LAUREL'S
KITCHEN
CARING

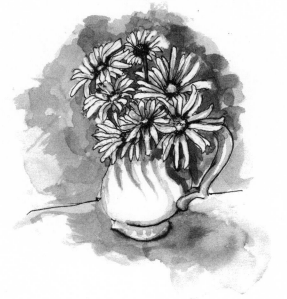

LAUREL'S KITCHEN
Caring

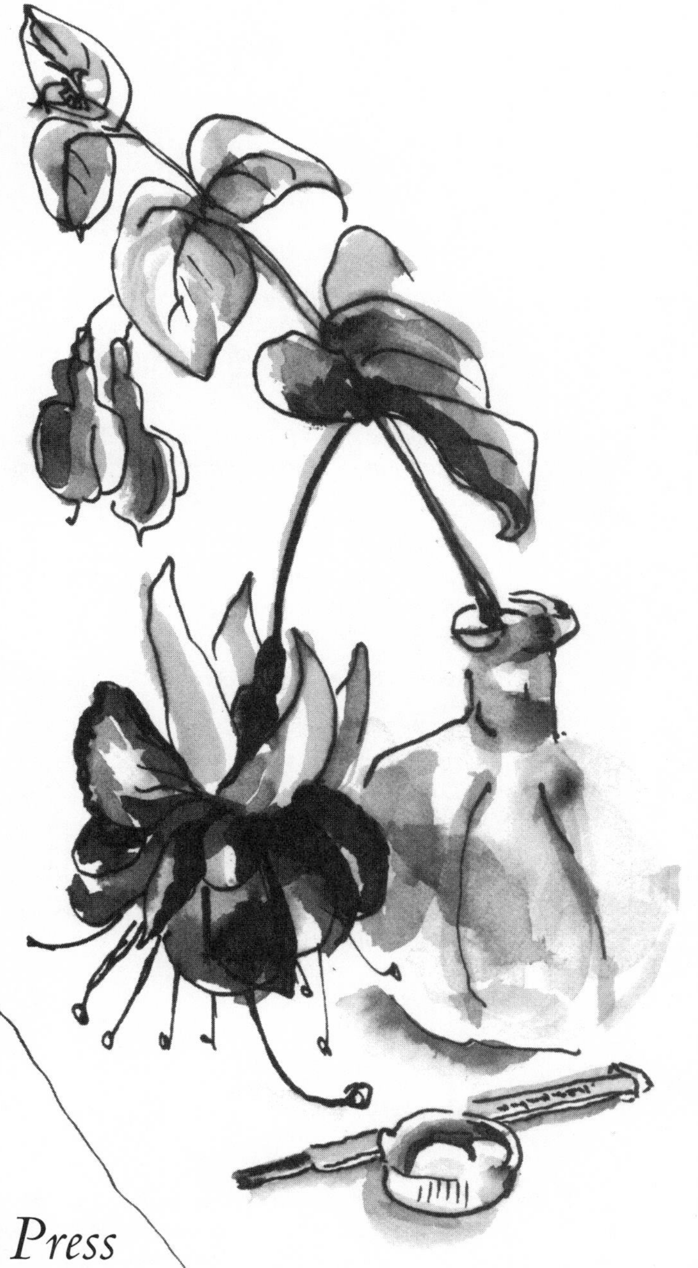

*Recipes for
Everyday
Home
Caregiving*

*by Laurel Robertson
with Carol Lee Flinders &
Brian Ruppenthal, R.D.*

Ten Speed Press

THIS BOOK IS DEDICATED TO CHRISTINE

©1997 by The Blue Mountain Center of Meditation, Inc.
Illustrations ©1997 by Laurel Robertson
Cover illustration ©1997 by Ilka Jerabek

TEN SPEED PRESS
Post Office Box 7123
Berkeley, California 94707

Library of Congress Cataloging-in-Publication Data

Robertson, Laurel.

    Laurel's kitchen caring : whole-food recipes for everyday home caregiving / by Laurel Robertson, with Carol Lee Flinders & Brian Ruppenthal.
        p.   cm.
    Includes index.
    ISBN 0–89815–951–2 (pbk.)
      1. Cookery for the sick. 2. Home care services   I. Flinders, Carol.
II. Ruppenthal, Brian. III. Title
RM219.R63   1997
641.5′631–dc21   97–22618   CIP

Printed in Canada

1 2 3 4 5 6 7 8 9 10   03 02 01 00 99 98 97

CAUTIONARY NOTE The recipes, instructions, and nutritional information contained in this book are in no way intended as a substitute for medical counseling. Please do not attempt self-treatment of a medical problem without consulting a physician.

Table of Contents

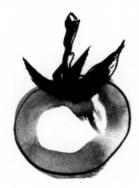

ACKNOWLEDGMENTS

Sarah, Diana, Gale, Sumner, Mark, Sandra, DiQ

Penelope & Tom; Julia

TESTERS
Rose, Gale O'Brien,
Chuck Cockelreas & Lynn Johnson
Mary Cormier, Maud Gleason, Sarah Harling
Julie MacLean, K.C. & Pamela Swartzel
Terry Wolfinger

Natasha Gorbitenko; Elise Stone

Sultana
Sylvia
Melissa
JoAnne
Mom & Daddy

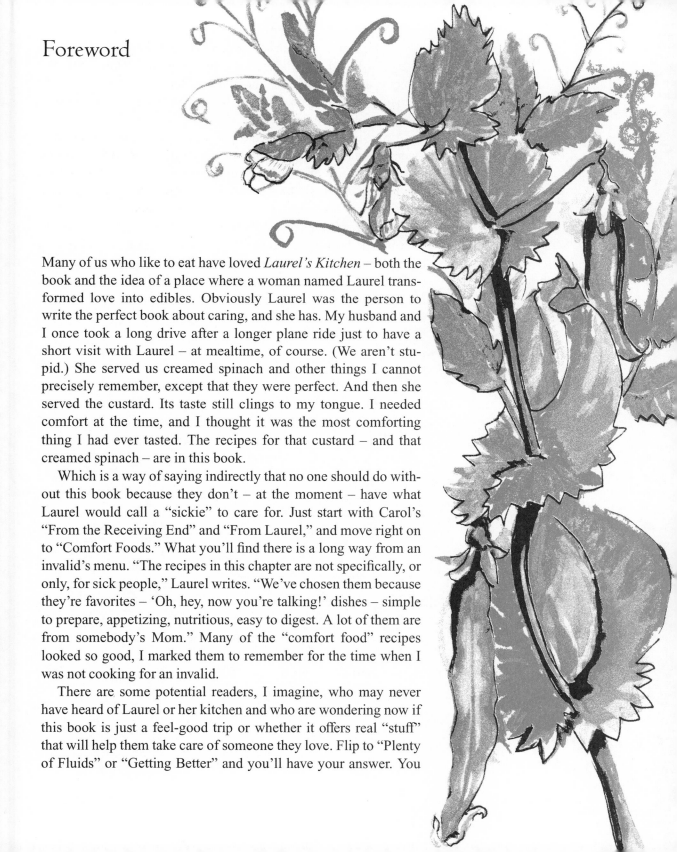

Foreword

Many of us who like to eat have loved *Laurel's Kitchen* – both the book and the idea of a place where a woman named Laurel transformed love into edibles. Obviously Laurel was the person to write the perfect book about caring, and she has. My husband and I once took a long drive after a longer plane ride just to have a short visit with Laurel – at mealtime, of course. (We aren't stupid.) She served us creamed spinach and other things I cannot precisely remember, except that they were perfect. And then she served the custard. Its taste still clings to my tongue. I needed comfort at the time, and I thought it was the most comforting thing I had ever tasted. The recipes for that custard – and that creamed spinach – are in this book.

Which is a way of saying indirectly that no one should do without this book because they don't – at the moment – have what Laurel would call a "sickie" to care for. Just start with Carol's "From the Receiving End" and "From Laurel," and move right on to "Comfort Foods." What you'll find there is a long way from an invalid's menu. "The recipes in this chapter are not specifically, or only, for sick people," Laurel writes. "We've chosen them because they're favorites – 'Oh, hey, now you're talking!' dishes – simple to prepare, appetizing, nutritious, easy to digest. A lot of them are from somebody's Mom." Many of the "comfort food" recipes looked so good, I marked them to remember for the time when I was not cooking for an invalid.

There are some potential readers, I imagine, who may never have heard of Laurel or her kitchen and who are wondering now if this book is just a feel-good trip or whether it offers real "stuff" that will help them take care of someone they love. Flip to "Plenty of Fluids" or "Getting Better" and you'll have your answer. You are dialoguing here with someone who has been there. There are ideas for liquid diets, ideas for pepping up or cooling down the touchy digestive system, ideas for adding calories when your patient needs to put on weight. (Badly needed ideas in the midst of a culture obsessed with dieting.)

Your standard "health care providers," as Laurel points out, went to school and got degrees because they wanted to help sick people. The rest of us, who thought we had other more important things to do, usually find ourselves cast unexpectedly in the role of caretaker for someone who needs our ministrations. Fitting time to care into schedules that labor-saving technology seems to have made busier is a stress. The process of taking care can't be done "efficiently," only lovingly – or impatiently. So even as she tells you what you can do to help, Laurel will forgive you for your resentment at being thrown unasked into the caregiver role, empathize with your lapses of courage, and help you feel better about your losses of patience.

Those of us who cook for ourselves and others are in one sense always health care providers, which means this is a book to have on your shelf wherever you presently find yourself. And that brings me to the issue of compromise. Most of us, by adulthood, have developed strong ideas about what we eat and don't eat. I myself try always to eat seasonally and locally and mostly eat what I grow – which means no peaches or asparagus in December. Others can't get through the day without a banana, believe passionately in the necessity of bagels, are convinced of the evils of sugar, or butter or soft drinks or meat or . . . Caring is about bringing comfort to someone who may not share your tastes or your prejudices – especially in ill health. Caring is about loving that person enough to buy and prepare things you would otherwise not have in your kitchen.

When you read this book, you will see that Laurel knows all caring is local and specific. She will cheer you on when you do whatever it takes to make your patient feel comforted. The book is meant, as she says, to be a loving letter from a friend. And a friend is someone who never makes you feel inadequate, but wholeheartedly sings your praises for doing your caring best.

JOAN GUSSOW, ED.D.
Professor emeritus of Nutrition and Education, Teachers College, Columbia University; author, lecturer, and passionate vegetable grower.

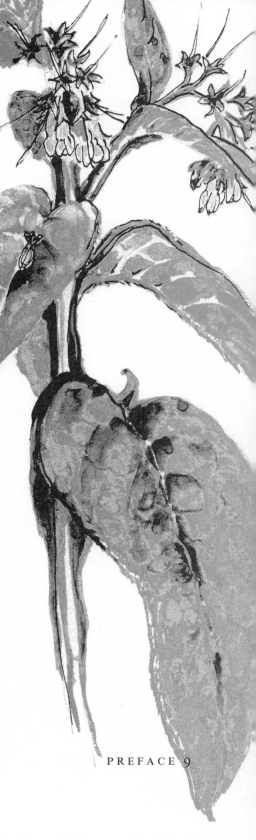

From the Receiving End

When Laurel asked me to write a preface to the *Caring* book I didn't think I had anything in particular to contribute, beyond recalling for her the heart-shaped pieces of toast with strawberry jam that my mother brought me when I was five and had rheumatic fever – one of the few instances I can recall when anybody has had to try to tempt my appetite.

Then, something happened. It didn't have anything directly to do with food, but it left me feeling that maybe I do indeed have something to add.

It was late, for me, on a Wednesday night early in October. I had given a talk at a public library an hour's drive from our home. Most of the drive home was along gently curving country highways. A lovely, soporific sort of drive. You probably see what's coming. I wish I had. I'd never given much thought to the dangers of falling asleep at the wheel, and didn't catch the warning signs. I nodded off just as I was heading down the last hill, a hundred feet from our driveway. My nervous system must have said, "There – we're home" and let go.

We'll pass over what took place over the next twenty or thirty seconds – especially since I'll never really know what took place, except that the part I was awake for was as frightening as anything I can remember ever. The upshot was that my car was beyond repair, and while I wasn't, I was going to need some time, some medical attention, and, for a couple of months, a certain amount of care.

It was clever of me to have run amok at exactly the place I did, because immediate care was close at hand. Within minutes, members of the volunteer fire department were there – men I knew, who couldn't have been more solicitous and skilled – and within a few minutes more, my husband's brother Rick, a physician, who lives just a mile from us. Rick rode with me in the ambulance and helped me get settled in at the hospital.

I'm sure I was scared, and I was in pain, but what I remember – and even at the time, I think this is what I was most conscious of – is the incredible tenderness that one person after another extended. Tenderness that was not just solace, but kept creatively figuring out things that helped. My elbow was broken, for example, so it would have made sense to cut my long-sleeved dress away, but when I grimaced (it was a brand new dress!) the emergency room nurse worked with me – and it took some doing – to get it off intact. As she scrubbed away at my face to clean it up before my son saw it, I remember thinking I felt like a kitten being rough-licked by its mother. Later that night after the X rays, another nurse helped bed me down. I was pretty well medicated by this time, and sleepy, but the pain in my back was real, and again I remember thinking as she molded pillows around me, supporting my back and legs so I could rest, What a genius this woman is! How does she know to do what she is doing? Do they teach this?

And really, that impression never altered the whole five days I was hospitalized.

In fact, though, the hospital staff could only do so much. When you've been ill or injured, and you can't take care of yourself, there are things that hospitals, doctors, and nurses really can't do for you – that only family and friends can do. Things that have to do with long and intimate association – with people knowing what means comfort to you, and security, and ease.

Food is an exceedingly important case in point. I can't remember a single bite of hospital food – can't even remember what was on the trays. Nothing. I do recall that every morning someone presented me with the hospital menu and asked me to check off what sounded good. I remember looking blankly at the form and checking every box relating to fruit – fresh fruit, fruit juice, fruit yogurt. But as to actually eating? I couldn't do it. Not until food started flowing in from home: Spanakopita, delicate pasta dishes, an exquisite fruit tart from friends who run a notable bakery; light soups. Food prepared by people who knew what I love to eat.

One hears such horror stories about hospital food, and they are so unfair. When you're levelled by pain (to say nothing of painkillers, tranquilizers and muscle relaxants), your need is for the absolutely familiar – and that's going to be different for everyone. No dietitian can be expected to provide that. There are places in the world where when someone is hospitalized, the family comes along, to do the cooking and caring, and I can really see the therapeutic value in that. When JoAnne walked in with that Spanakopita, still warm from the oven, it tasted of home and affection as well as fresh spinach, and I almost inhaled it, and I know it made me stronger.

I think I'm closing in now on what it is I want to say – what it is I've actually learned this past few months. It has to do with one's vitality, one's "life force," and its relationship to the recuperative process. Recovering from an injury takes all the energy you've got – the less you must spend on anything else, the better. Best of all is when friends and family are there, close at hand, and they want to help and do, creatively, so that you can give yourself over completely to the healing process. I've just had the privilege of experiencing this, and I can't say enough about how beneficial it is.

With a back injury and a broken elbow, there were so many things I couldn't do for myself. That could have been deeply distressing, but by the time I got home – still in a pharmaceutical fogbank – someone seemed to have anticipated every need. A collective someone, as it turned out. My bed was piled high with extra pillows, and there was a reclining chair I'd never seen before; the bathtub had been fitted with a handhold and seat, and I had a long "pincer" to pick things up with so I wouldn't try to bend over. Every morning Gale would drop by to help me bathe and dress, and every few days someone would come by to change my sheets. Another friend who's been studying herbal medicine showed up every night. Her three-year-old would help her apply a warm comfrey poultice to my back while her five-year-old played on the reclining chair. I was home now, and the food from our community's kitchen was just what I craved: fresh, organic vegetables, simply but deliciously cooked; good, honest, whole-grain bread, great soups, cereals, and fruits. Every day, it seemed, somebody would think of something to make life easier for me and my family, and most amazing of all, it was all so freely and happily given.

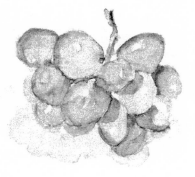

Once I realized that I could really just let go – that even my attachment to clean cotton sheets was being indulged – I did. I slept long and well, without anxiety. Gratitude and trust became a pretty much continuous state of mind. I healed rapidly.

Before, I hadn't even begun to understand what an enormous and powerful gift that kind of attention can be. Now I think about it a lot, and the laughter and camaraderie of helper and helped. I remember my pain, but I remember much more the eager readiness of my friends to alleviate it in every way imaginable. I know my turn will come, as everyone's does, to be on the other side of the equation. So I'm immensely grateful to Laurel for compiling so much of what she knows into the Caring book.

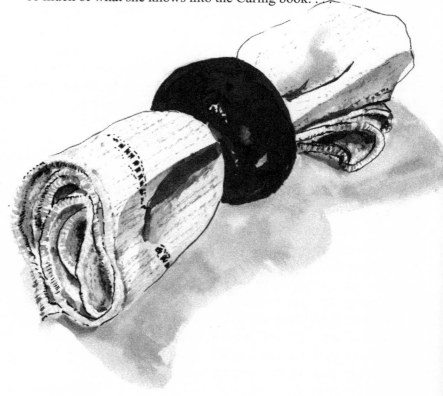

From Laurel

On top of the pile of papers in the back corner of my desk is a yellowed newspaper clipping. I haven't figured out where to put it, so it keeps getting buried and resurfacing – but that's OK, I like reading it again. The reporter is talking with people who have returned to life after having died, in medical terms. The interviewees tell how at the time of their "death" they experienced once again all the events of their life, including all their mistakes. The thing that's so interesting to me is that even their worst blunders don't oppress them – what they regret is the opportunities they had to show love that they let slip by. *Opportunities to show love,* a woman says, *are life's real treasures.*

Treasures. This book is for claiming treasures, big and small. Sparkling little gems – you nab them now and then. A friend has the flu, and you stop by with flowers, a funny story, a jar of broth – both of you get a bright memory to keep. Glorious treasures – crown-jewels magnitude – well, chances for them come along too. Then, love asks for more, and caring may span days and weeks, may put the rest of your life on hold. Is anyone ever prepared for that? But there it is, and prepared or not, we want to do all we can.

In the past several years, because of sad events, I have been privileged to watch some fine caregivers in action. This little book hopes to carry their spirit to people who have these precious opportunities, and want to give their best. During this time my own behind-the-lines contribution has been the Kitchen Patrol, and so here you have recipes, some of my own, and some from friends, ranging from comforting dishes for childhood snuffles and grumps, to real-food subsistence for people who are so ill they find it hard to eat at all.

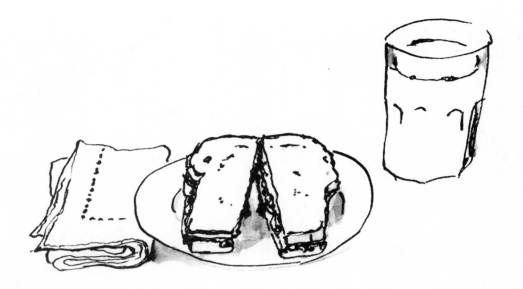

It is a closely guarded secret these days, but home-prepared food – "from scratch" or not – *is best*. This is so because of what motivates the cook. I admit that sometimes you and I, working at the stove, might not always be in the greatest mood – but even then, we posses a magic unknown to Burger Bell or Chez Aubergine. I claim that we home cooks have nothing less than a sacred flame burning on our heart's hearth. It lights what we think of, what we aim for, what we cook – what we, better than anyone, *know*, and that is how best to nourish these particular dear people who come to sit around our table. No chef or corporation knows how Ari likes his pancakes, or what gets Chris to eat a pile of broccoli. They can't take into consideration what kind of a day Sandy had, how hot and smoggy it is, or even that, out in the garden, the first brussels sprouts are ready, and some dumb snail took a nibble out of Mimi's really huge tomato. We, you and I, do know all that, and more. And it all goes into our stew when we fix a meal, and *that* is what makes home cooking utterly different and utterly, incomparably better – even when everyone is healthy.

But, when one of them gets sick! *Then* your loving savvy, your personalized touches, make *such* a difference. We aren't talking fussy – your sure aim is what counts, not how much time you put in. The recipes in this book cook up quick and easy. There's plenty else to do when you're taking care of someone, besides spending a lot of extra time in the kitchen.

ABOUT THOSE "CROWN JEWELS"...

There we are, hurtling through life. How hard it is to think about staying in with someone who is sick, maybe just sitting in the silence with them, sharing hours, pain, maybe death. I don't remember having been aware of anyone's doing this kind of thing when I was growing up – well, when my Grandpa was sick, there was a lady who came to help out. Her name was Bertha Hartley. The grown-ups said to each other in low voices that she was an angel and the family was so fortunate to have her come. I think maybe she was a retired nurse. What she did was go to a family where someone was dying. She would stay with them, sleep on the couch, and give such loving care, for days or weeks or months – sort of a one-woman travelling hospice. I was a preteen then, and it seemed to me a most amazing way to live. I wondered, did she even have a home of her own? Did she ever have any fun? But I recognized that Bertha seemed confident, admirably competent, and happier than other grown-ups. She certainly was never at a loss about what to do with her time. Nor ever wanted anything from anyone, either.

"Your health care providers" went to school, worked hard, and got degrees and certificates because they knew they wanted to help sick people. You and I find ourselves in caregiving roles seemingly by accident, and maybe we ask ourselves, Why me? But when you think about it, at some time or other *everyone* gets sick, and so anyone who has friends or family (fairly universal) will be a caregiver perforce, sooner or later. Naturally, once we find ourselves there, we want to do a good job.

Safe to say, it's never easy. There is the rest of your life. There is your lack of experience – you aren't always sure what to do. You feel anxiety about your sickie, and there are other pressures too. But – I have this from a doctor! – no professional can supply what you have to offer. Your personalized, loving care helps the healing process in so many ways. *It can help you too.* A hard school. Let it teach you to slow down, to focus; to know what is really important. To learn, wonderfully, the kind of tough tenderness that enables you to remain sunny when your charge is irritable because of pain. "You know they don't mean to be unpleasant," says a friend who works as a hospice volunteer, "They can't help it. When you remain calm and smiling, it helps them so much. They really appreciate it, though they won't be able to tell you so at the time. Oftentimes, they do tell me so, later

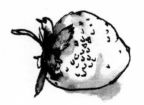

on." Penelope says, "I felt I had grown a foot taller the day I realized, *I don't have to win this argument.*"

Practicing caring opens your own deeper creativity, so that you can keep coming up with something new to try, and give each new plan your enthusiasm. And keep coming up with little comforts – improvised custom pillows or yet another funny story – that make life better for both of you. Maybe hardest is learning to stay detached enough to be able to step back and see what is needed, maybe something entirely different from what you have been doing up till now. Or to see when you yourself are falling into a negative state of mind, in time to take steps to restore your mental buoyancy. No one starts out knowing how to do all this – one caregiving friend laughs ruefully: "We learn by error and trial."

Mahatma Gandhi said he would have liked to have been a nurse. *Not me!* I scored about zero on "social service" in my Career Aptitude Test in high school – but I have gotten interested. Sharing caregiving duties with friends has let us know and trust each other in a deep and relaxed way that no other context could have done. Giving and receiving care, and being around some very special caregivers who have been able to hang in there with such love through demanding days and months of illness – well, now I can see that this is an unmatched school for goodness: for learning patience by practicing it; endurance, by toughing it through; for learning to love more and better under fire; for discovering big-time the joy of giving. I am beginning to understand why Gandhi said that.

What we give is so much more than a meal, or a bath, or a backrub. To some extent, every illness poses the question, *Am I worth being taken care of?* By the willing care we give, we answer, *Yes!!* But even the best care isn't more than a holding pattern until the patient is ready to get well; then the answer surges from within, *Yes! My life is worthwhile!* – then the real healing begins. We caregivers, we try to love and to give always with our whole heart, but never to miss any chance to pass the reins to the patient. Never create emotional dependency, selfish attachment on either side. The object is to end up with *two* healthy people.

ॐ

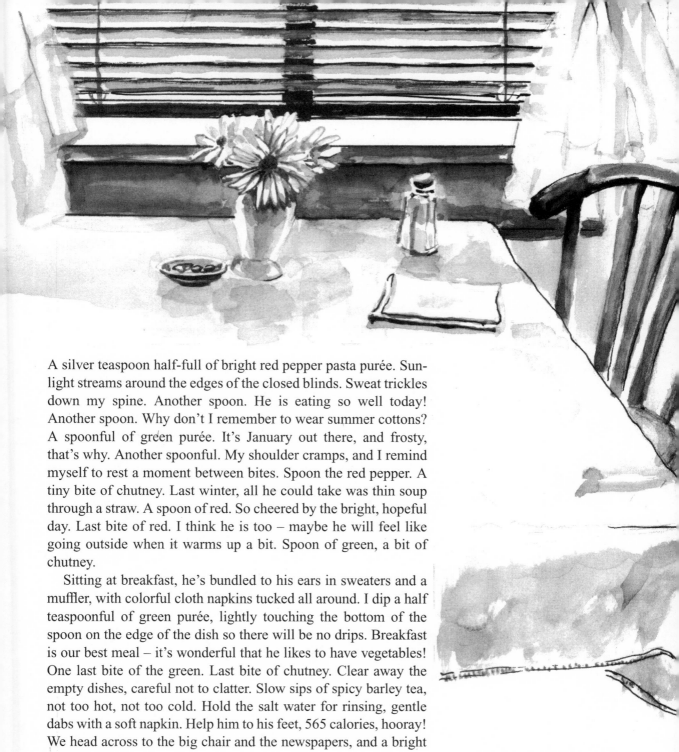

A silver teaspoon half-full of bright red pepper pasta purée. Sunlight streams around the edges of the closed blinds. Sweat trickles down my spine. Another spoon. He is eating so well today! Another spoon. Why don't I remember to wear summer cottons? A spoonful of green purée. It's January out there, and frosty, that's why. Another spoonful. My shoulder cramps, and I remind myself to rest a moment between bites. Spoon the red pepper. A tiny bite of chutney. Last winter, all he could take was thin soup through a straw. A spoon of red. So cheered by the bright, hopeful day. Last bite of red. I think he is too – maybe he will feel like going outside when it warms up a bit. Spoon of green, a bit of chutney.

Sitting at breakfast, he's bundled to his ears in sweaters and a muffler, with colorful cloth napkins tucked all around. I dip a half teaspoonful of green purée, lightly touching the bottom of the spoon on the edge of the dish so there will be no drips. Breakfast is our best meal – it's wonderful that he likes to have vegetables! One last bite of the green. Last bite of chutney. Clear away the empty dishes, careful not to clatter. Slow sips of spicy barley tea, not too hot, not too cold. Hold the salt water for rinsing, gentle dabs with a soft napkin. Help him to his feet, 565 calories, hooray! We head across to the big chair and the newspapers, and a bright new day.

Sometimes a patient has something more than the usual cold or flu, maybe an illness that makes it difficult to chew, or to take solid food. The chapter "Getting Better" offers recipes for foods that are nourishing, tasty, exceptionally easy to eat and digest – thin soups, purées, and soft foods, with many suggestions for adjusting the nutrition in different directions for different needs, from sickness through to health.

Cooking like this won't ever make the food pages of the newspaper, nor did you, or we, ever hope to face such a wrenching situation. Still, we whose caring includes cooking have the chance to make these hard times a feast of love – even if, or maybe *because* the cuisine is itself perforce so bleak. Now is when our imagination and compassion team up to find ways to make the meals as appealing as they can be. Sure, you aren't trained in nutrition, but that won't stop you from finding out how your efforts can make things better. What particular foods agree especially well? Are there some things, or some preparation methods, to avoid? Might some even contribute to the cure? If certain foods are beneficial, how many different ways can you cook them to keep mealtime interesting? Take asparagus – one exceptionally nutritious and digestible food. Well, so there's asparagus soup, mousse, pudding, timbale, aspic, crepes, pasta, soufflé, ravioli, quiche, patties, *somosas, Chinoise, tiropita,* and – oh yeah – spears. Not only great chefs are artists!

I'm the last one to claim that this sort of cooking is a bunch of fun and frolic. Lots of days there are tears in the soup, and lots of days you're there in the kitchen when you might otherwise be walking on the beach. Your patient, and your aspirin bottle, are losing weight, but *you* are definitely not . . .

And yet, and yet. Caring for someone is one of the rare, real things we can do in this life. It is hard. But wouldn't you expect an intensely creative activity to be hard? Some good times, some terrible ones, some boring ones, some scary ones. Some hours when your endurance is tested beyond what you ever thought you could survive. Times when you come up with a solution to a problem quickly, other times when nothing seems to work though you try everything you can think of, and more. But what you are doing is greater art than painting a masterpiece, or writing a sonata, because it is, most of all, *you* that you are crafting as you tenderly care for your friend; very likely you find depths in yourself you never suspected were there.

Hold tight to your sense of humor. Resist courageously when your mind tries to convince you you are wasting your time, not doing a good job, worth more than this, going to have a nervous breakdown, etc., and all the other weasely scenarios our lower self uses to bring us down. Learning to recognize them is an education in itself. Patiently to overcome them, and to keep on helping even when it's hard, is better than college. Afterward, life opens to a different perspective, and very likely you have grown closer to your real self – a happier, kinder, wiser, and more peaceful person than before.

There are some things this book is not. It is not a nursing man-

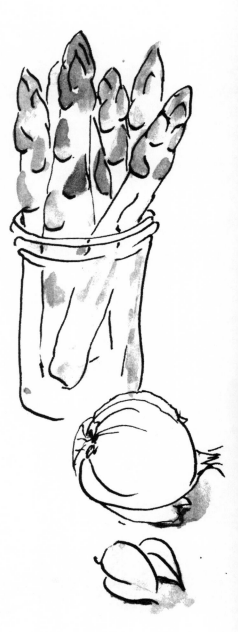

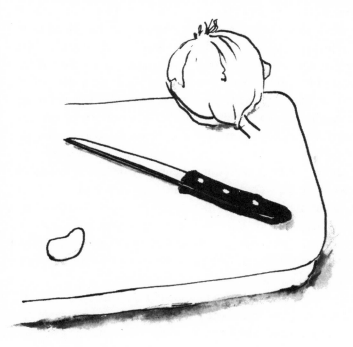

ual – there is no medical information here. The book is not about prevention – there are "healthy" recipes in it, but our emphasis is on addressing problems, balancing needs in unusual situations. Schooled in the whole-foods – low-fat paradigm of the *Laurel's Kitchen* books, it's been boggling for us to adjust to the idea that *sometimes,* yes, a patient needs extra calories so much that cooking with extra fat is OK, even necessary! And *sometimes,* yes, a person *does* need extra protein; sometimes, less fiber. We have tried to let you see how you can tailor any recipe's preparation or ingredients to your patient's particular needs.

You who share our passion that food is best when it is locally grown and fresh may be astonished to see so many recipes for asparagus, for example, which is in season so briefly. All I can say is, when someone very dear is very sick, if only asparagus appeals, asparagus it is, wherever it was grown – how fortunate that it's something so nutritious and digestible. (When you cook for someone in this situation, you do make a mental note about what a blessing it is to have learned to enjoy a wide variety of nutritious foods, so that the strait of illness isn't narrowed further by rigid likes and dislikes!)

This book has no recipes containing meat. If you're not a vegetarian, you might wonder whether it would suit you, whether our recipes would suit anyone you know who's sick. Our friend Lois is a nurse of many years' experience – shall I tell you what she says? People who are sick usually want, and manage best with, simple and pure foods, foods with a clear clean taste, like fruit. They often will ask for dishes they remember their mother having given them when they were little. This book is full of such wholesome, comforting food, good food for anyone to eat, easy to digest.

The recipes can be prepared inexpensively because they don't depend on packaged commercial products, just normal basics from the supermarket and the natural foods store. If you grow your own vegetables, or if fresh, organically grown produce is available to you, these offer particular benefits to a body fighting to get well, whether the problem is a little cold or flu, or a serious long-term illness.

I think you'll find much here that is helpful. I hope that we can be good company, too, and cheer you on during what can be a trying, and a lonely, time. Maybe think of this little volume as a loving letter from a friend. If you have helpful suggestions from your own caregiving experience, write and let us share them.

Comfort Foods

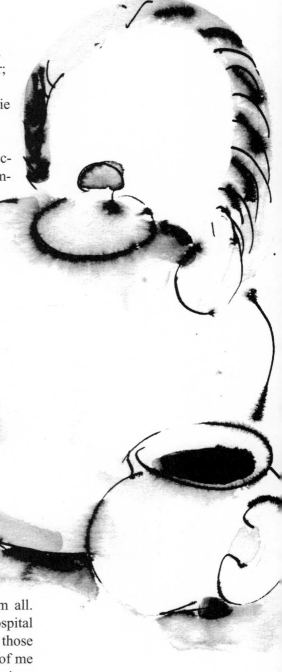

Graduation! Good-bye, roommates' jabbering radios; adiós, neglected coffee cups; so long, pounding on the shower door; farewell, waiting to use the phone; adieu, struggling for Cleanup Fairness! At last I reign over my very own little aerie of an apartment – my own phone, my own shower, my own (hooray!) kitchen … Heaven. Right. Well, two lonely, blue November days into a wretched, stuffy flu and I'm having second thoughts. Dark, cold windows dripping, sleety rain drumming, dysfunctional radiator clanging but stone cold. Cold walls, cold lumpy pillow, cold, lonely, miserable, melancholy heart – abandoned, forlorn, forgotten . . .

But what? A knock?

Ta-Daa! Enter: beautiful Carol, laughing, with a loaded tray: steaming minestrone soup, hot toast, and, oh, most wonderful, a big bowl of her special honey custard. (Sunshine, flowers, birds singing.)

You never forget something like that.

A friend says, What do you *mean* "Comfort Food"?

꒰ Bethann was in the hospital for a week. Friends brought her flasks of Golden Noodle Soup, little casseroles, homemade muffins, yogurt pie. She cherished them all. "My body was too sick to eat anything but the blandest hospital food, but some other vital nourishment was coming from all those wonderful things people had brought. I kept them in front of me and just looked at them. That fed me in some other, mysterious way."

As I write this, Jim is dying of AIDS. Sylvia has cared for him for almost two years. She says his time is coming to an end, but maybe he will hold on till Christmas, a few more days. He eats only fruit now. *How do you give it to him?* "Well, if it is an orange, I peel it and break it into the sections and put them on a plate. Grapes, I wash and pull off the stems. He can enjoy a variety of kinds of fruit – he even had watermelon last week, you know, cut into bite-size pieces." *Watermelon and grapes in December,* I am thinking. But Sylvia looks up, with a different expression. "Now he says if he had more time left, he would want to spend it just helping people, just helping, any way, any way he could."

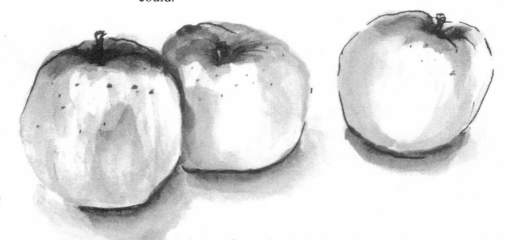

Carol was five when she had rheumatic fever. Her mom worked hard to tempt her appetite. Carol remembers toast painstakingly cut into heart shapes, spread with cream cheese and raspberry jam.

Comfort food. The food is a part of it, maybe the vehicle, so to say, for something else that is mysteriously, powerfully, healing. I conducted a small survey: what is Comfort Food to you? Mostly people would look into the distance and then smile suddenly, remembering something their mom used to make for them when they were small. "My mom used to arrange orange half-slices in a sunburst around a little pile of powdered sugar." Never anything fancy – foods of childhood, simple dishes with clear tastes. Applesauce. Oatmeal with brown sugar. Toast triangles. Hot soup. Buttered noodles. Plain vegetables with salt and pepper. Tapioca pudding. Fruit cup.

If you are caring for a close family member, you probably know what to give them without thinking much about it. Otherwise, take this idea from a friend who does home nursing: She says some people have never paid a bit of attention to food, so that even when hungry, they may not have the foggiest idea what would taste good to them. She'll sit down with them, and together they leaf through a cookbook, tagging the pages with recipes that sound appealing.

❧

The recipes in this chapter are not specifically, or only, for sick people. We've chosen them because they're favorites – "Oh, hey, now you're talking!" dishes – simple to prepare, appetizing, nutritious, easy to digest. A lot of them are from somebody's Mom.

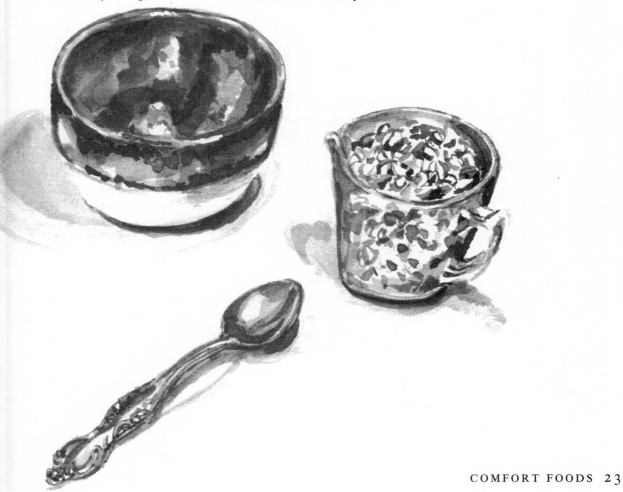

Kid Pleasers

These are not for dire times, but for sniffles and grumps, when life gives us lumps.

❧ *Toast Triangles:* Top crisp toast with honey or jam, with cream cheese, shake-cheese, or a sprinkle of cinnamon and sugar. For young ones, remove crusts. Cut the toast piece corner-to-corner twice to make four small triangles.

❧ *Honey-milk:* A mug of steaming milk with a spoon of honey stirred in, maybe topped with a dash of nutmeg. Especially effective when offered while one is snugly tucked into a cocoon of pillows and blankets.

❧ *Milk Toast:* Cut or break freshly made toast into bite-size pieces and put them in a bowl. Cover with milk and eat at once. Some will want sweetener.

❧ *Slow Toast:* Lightly butter airy whole wheat bread, and cut into strips, discarding crusts. Arrange strips across a cake-cooling rack, and bake at 325°F until completely crisp – the time will vary, roughly half an hour. Bread that contains dairy products browns quickly. To be sure it dries out completely you may need to lower the oven temperature and allow more time, because Slow Toast is best if delicately golden rather than brown.

❧ *Mom's special-occasion cinnamon toast:* Toast slices of bread on one side under the broiler. Meantime, mix ¼ teaspoon cinnamon and a tablespoon sugar per slice. Butter the untoasted side of the bread and spread with the sugar and cinnamon mixture. Carefully put back under the broiler, watching vigilantly. As soon as the top is bubbly, take toast out, and put it on a plate. Allow to cool a little bit before serving.

❧ *Potato Pancakes:* "Building" food. Good with fruit cup and maybe scrambled eggs. For robust convalescents, serve alongside steamed broccoli florets and red-ripe tomatoes or fresh salsa. (More potato recipes on pages 36–39.)

❧ *Softies:* Steam potato, then peel, salt, and mash roughly. (Leftover potatoes work nicely.) Drop spoonfuls on a medium-hot buttered griddle; turn when golden brown on the bottom. Brown on the other side, and serve.

❧ *Puffies*: Steam and mash a big potato, and salt to taste. Beat an egg and stir it in. Add grated cheese or cottage cheese, if wanted. Cook as above.

❧ *Crusties:* Grate raw potato and *rinse with plenty of cold water;* drain. Sprinkle with salt, and drop on oiled, medium-hot griddle, turning when nicely brown. Reduce heat somewhat, and cook until tender. (This one takes a little longer. But even if you make it with only the tiniest bit of oil on a nonstick griddle, it comes out crispy and delectable.)

❧ *Cotters:* Freeze whole ripe apricots or blueberries, strawberries, raspberries, seedless grapes. Mini-popsicles to pass out in tiny paper cups, or on oversize toothpicks for older children.

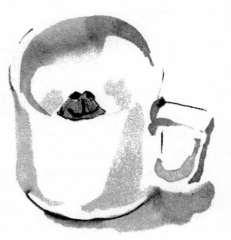

❧ Special, and soothing to a sore throat: "Popsicles" made by freezing fruit juice. For *"creamsicles"* mix a spoonful of orange juice concentrate with mild yogurt and a few drops of vanilla. Freeze in small paper cups or popsicle forms or in nonmetal ice cube trays using oversized toothpicks as sticks. (No normal-size toothpicks for young children, for safety.)

❧ *Bubbly:* For convalescing schoolkids, mix fruit juice with carbonated mineral water 1:3.

❧ Smoothies are soothing, nourishing, and a mom-certified remedy for the grumps – turn to page 152–153.

Add a handful of alphabet noodles to any soup or broth when preparing it for a child.

See also, the comforting sweets at the end of the chapter.

Old-Fashioned Pancakes

2 cups whole wheat flour–
coarse stone-ground flour
much preferred here
(½ cup wheat germ or ses-
ame seeds, etc.)
2 teaspoons baking powder
1 tablespoon brown sugar
1 teaspoon salt

2 large eggs (½ cup)
2½ to 3 cups fresh milk

2 tablespoons oil

For us, this is *pancakes*. Can't beat 'em. If your flour is finely ground, including wheat germ, seeds, or bran, or some cornmeal, if possible, will make your pancakes lighter.

ॐ

Stir together all the dry ingredients.

Beat the eggs lightly and combine with the milk, then add to the dry ingredients and mix briefly. Stir in oil.

Heat the griddle. It should be hot enough so that when you sprinkle water drops on the surface, they dance. Unless the griddle is unseasoned, it shouldn't need any grease. Pour the batter onto griddle by large spoonfuls. Cook over medium heat, turning once when bubbles come to the surface and pop, and the edges are slightly dry.

Makes 18 pancakes. Batter stores fine in the refrigerator for a few days. If it darkens on top, that's OK – just stir it up and pour.

FANCIES
Before you pour the batter, sprinkle the griddle with ses-ame, sunflower, or poppy seeds.

PANCAKE MIX
Convenient at home, and a thoughtful gift to take to a caregiving friend.
Combine the dry ingredients for a few batches. Store air-tight in the refrigerator.
To reconstitute:
  1 cup dry mix
  1 egg
  1¼ cups milk
  1 tablespoon oil

VARIATIONS
Buttermilk Pancakes: Replace baking powder with 1 teaspoon baking soda and substitute buttermilk for milk. May need a little more liquid. Very tender pancakes.
Blueberry Pancakes: Ah. Add a cup of fresh blueberries to the batter or drop several on each cake after it is poured.
Fresh Corn Pancakes: Add a cup of cooked corn kernels.

TAILORING

Reduce the fat:
• Use 2 egg whites, or egg replacer, instead of the whole egg.
• Leave out the oil. This does change the character of the pancakes significantly, but with coarsely ground flour they can be tender and light. Cook oil-free pancakes longer, over slightly lower heat.

No dairy: Use the dry ingredients as listed, plus water in place of the egg and milk measure. Soymilk will work also. Here especially, using coarse flour makes better pancakes.

Oatmeal Pancakes

Oatmeal Pancakes have received much more than their share of fan mail. Very satisfying stackers, good even plain.

৵

Combine the milk and rolled oats in a bowl and let stand at least 5 minutes.

Add the oil and beaten eggs, mixing well. Stir in the flour, sugar, baking powder, and salt. Mix just until the dry ingredients are moistened.

Bake on a hot, lightly oiled griddle, using ¼ cup of batter for each pancake. Turn them when the top is bubbly and the edges are slightly dry.

Makes 10 to 12 pancakes.

WHEATLESS OAT CAKES

Make 1¾ cups of flaky meal by spinning 2 cups or so of rolled oats in blender. Use instead of the combined oat and wheat measure. Mix ingredients and let stand about 5 minutes. If griddle is not well seasoned, oil it lightly, as these pancakes tend to stick.

Makes 12.

1¼ cups milk
1 cup rolled oats

1 tablespoon oil
2 eggs, beaten

½ cup whole wheat flour
1 tablespoon brown sugar
1 teaspoon baking powder
¼ teaspoon salt

Buckwheat Pancakes

Stir the dry ingredients together.

Add the oil, beaten egg, and milk, and mix briefly. Cook the pancakes on a medium-hot, lightly oiled griddle. Buckwheat pancakes take a little extra time to cook, so wait until bubbles appear all over the surface before turning them.

Makes 18 pancakes.

NOTE: To make fresh buckwheat flour from whole groats, put them in the blender (dry) and blend until they make flour.

1 cup buckwheat flour
2 teaspoons baking powder
1 cup whole wheat flour
½ teaspoon salt
1 tablespoon brown sugar

1 tablespoon oil
2 eggs, beaten
2 cups fresh milk
(grated peel of 1 orange)

Mother Leela's Rice

A friend from India says when she was small her mother always made this for her when she was under the weather, especially if she had a little diarrhea. Later, when she was in her teens, it soothed her menstrual cramps – Indian women know to avoid hot spices at those times, so this simple preparation is a favorite.

Now that she is a mom, she gives the same dish to her little boy. He eats it happily at those times when nothing else will do. Carol says, "Just reading this recipe, it's hard to tell how delicious it really is, particularly when you don't feel well."

≈

Start with hot, well-cooked rice. Stir in a little butter and a big spoonful of yogurt. No spices except salt. The yogurt will cool the hot rice so that it is just the right temperature.

If the patient is up to it, serve it with a little bit of green vegetable, like green beans or spinach, alongside.

Convalescent children for whom dairy products don't work welcome this dish made with coconut milk instead of the butter and yogurt.

1 tablespoon ghee or oil
(or less)
½ teaspoon black mustard
seeds*
an onion, chopped fine
(a green chili, chopped)
2 cups well-cooked rice
1 cup tart yogurt, to taste
salt to taste
(chopped coriander leaves)

VARIATION

Healthy eaters will enjoy zesty *Yogurt Rice:*
Heat the oil in a heavy skillet or saucepan. When it is hot but not yet smoking, drop in the seeds and cover the pan with a dry lid. The seeds will pop like popcorn. As soon as their popping noise diminishes slightly, add the onion, stir, and lower the heat. Keep stirring until the onion is translucent. Add the chopped chili, and continue to cook gently until the onion is soft. Stir in the rice, then add the yogurt. Garnish with coriander leaves.

*Black (or brown) mustard seeds are available in Indian stores. If this recipe sounds good to you but you don't have mustard seeds, omit them. A tasty substitute for their warmth of flavor in this recipe would be a sprinkle of toasted sesame seeds, added at the end.

Waffles

Waffles can be just the thing when you're sick. If you are a waffle fan, you have a favorite recipe – and if your patient is a family member it's probably her favorite, too! In that case, if her appetite needs prodding, no one else's recipe can match yours.

If you are a waffle fan, you will see right away that the following recipes are unusual – for one thing, they are innocent of waffles' normal hefty quantities of egg and butter. We have enjoyed them many, many times, however weird. Waffles for the adventurous, waffles that do not succumb to damp-sponge syndrome.

These recipes are our own tried-and-true versions of two of the creative waffle recipes in The Oats, Peas, Beans & Barley Cookbook, *by Edyth Young Cottrell (Woodbridge Press, 1989).*

Especially if you don't have a nonstick waffle iron, grease generously with lecithin spray. *Bake a full 8 minutes without lifting the lid.* If the lid resists opening, cook a couple of minutes more. Since the waffles take a while to bake, you may choose to prepare them ahead. Keep them warm for a little while on the rack in a 200°F oven (not stacked) – don't let them dry out, however.

Extras keep well in the refrigerator or freezer. Rewarm them in the toaster, or on the waffle iron.

Serve with either a sweet or savory topping. Makes a hearty dinner waffle with creamed spinach or curried vegetables.

Oat and Cashew Waffles

It's fun to share an old favorite. When Chuck tested this recipe, he wrote, "These were a real surprise. I didn't expect them to taste so good – nor that the texture would be so pleasant. A good alternate to rice crackers."

2¼ cups water
1½ cups rolled oats
⅓ cup raw cashews
1 tablespoon oil
½ teaspoon salt

In electric blender, spin all of the ingredients until light and foamy, about half a minute. Let stand while the waffle iron heats – the batter will thicken somewhat. Blend again, briefly, just before pouring.

Grease the waffle iron top and bottom with lecithin spray. Bake 8 to 10 minutes, until delicately brown. *(No peeking!)*

Makes 2 full 12″ × 6″ waffles.

For a homemade lecithin spray, see margin page 131.

Special Diets

Sarah went through a hard time when her asthma was aggravated by severe food allergies. I asked her what she learned that might help others who faced the need to begin a strict new diet. What she said is useful no matter what problem makes the changes necessary:

"I was self-conscious about eating different food until I realized that everybody always looks around to see what the other folks have on their plates – it probably goes back to our caveman days, when you had to check out what the other guy found, might be something good. Anyway, when I realized that, I stopped taking it personally.

"It is good to be very strict at first. For one thing, your cravings for particular things go away to some extent. Your health improves, which really makes you feel good about yourself. Later on, when you get less cautious and maybe aren't feeling very well, you remember how great you felt when you were being strict.

"Identify your 'trigger foods' – things you can't risk eating at all. Identify your personal 'comfort foods.' If they are forbidden, devise some substitute that works for you.

"If you really have to have something, buy only one – one cookie, not a box. A cone, not a pint. Late in the day, not early.

"Keep plenty of what you can eat on hand. Focus on the positive, be inventive, and give it the attention it needs.

"Plan ahead. Call the restaurant, for example. Most of them are happy to make a dish to your specifications.

"Avoid getting into untenable situations, where you are hungry when there is nothing around that's on your list.

"Once in a while, it may be worth having your treat and taking more medication, if you have that option. So much measuring and planning can make a person feel like a robot. But also it is good to remember when you are in a tight place, for example, at a party, you can fast. Keep food in its place.

"Talk with others who have similar problems, share ideas and support. But even with 'normal' people, remember that your self-discipline helps everyone who comes in contact with you. Everyone needs to improve their act, and your doing it inspires others. When you are in good control, you help others.

"Having a higher purpose in your life is the greatest help to prevent backsliding."

Stuart's Waffles

Stu perfected this recipe when Sarah was on a special diet. He made a big enough batch of these wheat-free, dairy-free, fat-free waffles "to satisfy three hungry eaters," plus extras to freeze. They are great popped into the toaster for another breakfast, and make a superior stand-in for bread. Sarah: "It was so great to have something we could all sit down and really enjoy together!"

Makes about 10 big waffles.

⁓

Soak the rice for 24 hours in about 8 cups of water. It will increase in volume to about 9 cups.

Soak the beans for 8 hours in 8 cups of water. They will swell to about 6 cups.

Strain the rice water into a bowl. Add water to the rice water to bring it up to 9 cups.

Discard water from beans and rinse them. Combine rice, rice water, beans, and salt, and blend them smooth in batches in blender, and transfer to a big bowl.

Let batter stand while the waffle iron heats on hottest setting. At the same time, preheat the oven to 325°F.

Use a nonstick waffle iron and spray lightly with lecithin spray before the first waffle. Bake waffles for *at least* 8 minutes. Use a timer! The red waffle light doesn't know about this kind of waffle. Take the waffle out, start the next, then put the first into the oven for about 5 minutes to finish cooking the soy, and to drive off some excess moisture.

From Stu:

Two waffle irons in parallel keep three eaters fed. I start a little ahead so there are batches in the oven when we begin to eat. I cook up the rest of the batter while I clean up after breakfast, setting the extras aside to freeze. They toast well.

6 cups brown rice
2¼ cups soy beans (or pinto beans for even lower fat)
1 tablespoon salt

You will need a nonstick pan and lecithin spray (e.g. Pam) – or the mixture described in the margin on page 131.

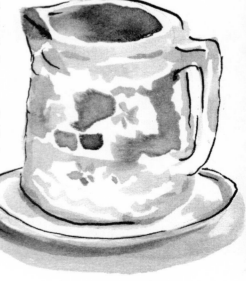

Crepes

1 cup milk or half water, half milk
¾ cup finely ground whole wheat flour
2 eggs or 3 whites
½ teaspoon salt

Nearly any child, ill or well, finds vegetables that have been rolled into a crepe infinitely more appealing than those which have not. Crepe batter takes no time to mix up, and keeps in the refrigerator, ready to use. Crepes are nutritious, and reliably provide an easy way to produce something jazzy quickly, using staples on hand. A culinary gold mine.

۶۰

DAIRY-FREE:
1 cup finely ground whole wheat flour
1½ cups water
½ teaspoon baking powder
½ teaspoon salt
1 tablespoon oil

Put all the ingredients together in a jar or blender and mix briefly, just until smooth. Let the batter stand for an hour or more, if you have the time. The batter should be thinner than pancake batter, thicker than half-and-half.

Blending the finely grated yellow peel of a lemon into the crepe batter gives the flavor a lift – especially nice in the nondairy and the low-fat versions.

Use a crepe pan, a 7″ skillet with sloped sides, or a griddle you can pick up and turn. Nonstick pans or seasoned iron ones work best. A quick squirt with lecithin spray or a touch of oil or butter between pours is usually all that is needed to prevent sticking.

Heat the pan over medium-high flame. Pour a scant ¼ cup of batter on the pan, then tilt and turn so the batter spreads into a thin, even circle. As soon as the top becomes visibly dry – less than a minute if they're thin – turn the crepe, and brown it lightly on the other side. If your crepes seem too thick, stir a little more liquid into the batter. Stack the crepes to fill later, or fill them as you go. The pretty, spotty side is the outside for a rolled crepe.

Makes about 12.

Crepe batter keeps in a jar in the refrigerator for days. It will darken a bit – that's OK. Just shake it up and proceed. Precooked, cooled crepes stacked on a plate, slipped into a plastic bag, keep for several days in the refrigerator; they also freeze well.

۶۰

A NOTE TO BEGINNERS

Learning to cook crepes is easy. You need a good pan like the one described above. Prepare a batch of batter and put it into a pitcher or measuring cup that has a pouring lip. Stir between pours. Give yourself permission to mess up as many as you need to – you'll be competent and confident before you use it up.

Some ideas for serving Crepes

✤ Creamed Spinach is the classic filling (see next page). With its intense flavor and outstanding nutrient content, spinach "justifies" the cream sauce. Other sauced vegetables work fine: asparagus cut small; broccoli; green beans and mushrooms. Ratatouille. Top the filled crepes with sauce or a sprinkle of Parmesan, or sliced tomatoes and chopped parsley. Bake, covered, just long enough to heat through.

✤ *Crepe Cake:* Stack crepes on a lightly oiled heatproof plate, alternating them with layers of cooked, thinly cut, nicely seasoned broccoli, greens, or asparagus, plus cottage and/or other favorite cheese; then salsa or chutney. Aim for harmonious flavors – cottage cheese with cheddar, broccoli, and spicy tomato salsa; or lightly creamed asparagus, cottage cheese, mango chutney. The vegetables should be salted unless the cheese is very salty. Spread the fillings evenly to keep the "cake" flat. Top with cheese and salsa, and bake long enough to melt the cheese inside. Cut and serve in wedges. Leftover wedges reheat just fine.

APPROXIMATELY:
9 crepes, more if you dare
2 cups sliced, cooked vegetables
1 cup salsa or chutney
2 cups cottage cheese

✤ Enchiladas Petaluma, page 57.

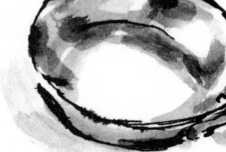

CREPES FOR DESSERT

✦ Fold crepes in quarters with warm marmalade.

✦ Fill them with cinnamon-laced applesauce, or stack with sliced fresh berries and honey yogurt (or whipped cream, sour cream, ricotta, yogurt cheese, you know); cut in wedges.

✦ For *German Pancakes,* squeeze a crepe with plenty of lemon juice and dust with powdered sugar, then roll tight and dust with more powdered sugar. Serve garnished with lemon wedges. A kid can eat a lot of these.

Easy Spinach Crepes

	FOR ONE *(3 crepes)*	FOR FOUR *(12 crepes)*
Cream sauce (heavy)	1 cup	4 cups
Spinach, cooked, squeezed well	⅔ cup	3 cups
Tiny peas (optional, but nice)	2–3 tablespoons	¼ –1 cup
Tiny cubes of jack or gruyere	1 tablespoon	¼ cup
Crepes	3	12

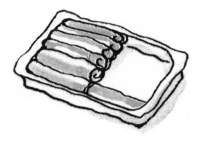

PREPARATION

Preheat oven to 350°F. Mix about ¾ of the cream sauce with the spinach, peas, and cheese. Check the salt and pepper, and adjust to taste. Use ⅓ cup of spinach mixture to fill each crepe, putting them seam-side down in a glass baking dish. (12 fit in 2 rows in a 9″ × 13″ pan.) Top with cream sauce and bake about 15 minutes, just long enough to heat through.

Crepes can be made in stages, the elements refrigerated before or after assembling, and before or after baking. If they are cold they take somewhat longer in the oven, of course.

ONE CUP (HEAVY)

3 tablespoons butter
3 tablespoons flour
   (we suggest whole wheat
   pastry flour)
1 cup of hot milk*
¼ teaspoon salt
(a pinch of nutmeg)

*You can use cold milk if you want to, but heating the milk helps prevent lumping.

CREAM SAUCE

Melt butter in a hefty pan over low flame. Stir in flour, cooking without browning for a minute. Add milk and bring to a boil, stirring all the while – use a wire whisk if you have one. Stir lumps smooth; if they persist, a brief spin in the blender will set things right. Add salt. Nutmeg is traditional.

⌁ *To reduce the fat:* Cut the butter down to one tablespoon per cup of skim or low fat milk. Quite acceptable flavorwise.

⌁ *A nonfat sauce that's not too bad:* Gently toast the flour in a dry pan, until it is fragrant but *not brown.* Add skim milk.

⌁ *No dairy:* Use oil instead of butter, plus grain milk or soymilk. We suggest that you add sautéed onion and/or mushrooms, and include the peas, to give flavor. Lower the baking temperature to 325F° to prevent too much browning when you use soymilk.

Blintzes

Delightful at any meal, variable as to calories. Serve with crushed berries or applesauce, and a dab of (nonfat) sour cream or yogurt.

Very good also made impromptu for the caregiving cook. Fill leftover crepes with cottage cheese and a dash of cinnamon, and eat them alongside some steaming hot greens, with applesauce if you have any.

Blintzes always make me think of Emily, a college friend, lovely and so ethereal, the first vegetarian I ever knew. I asked her to dinner, then remembered about her food and panicked – what could we serve? But my roommate Penny knew how to make blintzes, and we added broccoli spears, and fruit salad for dessert, and it was a big hit. Until then, it hadn't occurred to me that a person could survive without meat.

2 cups cottage cheese
1 tablespoon brown sugar
(1 tablespoon melted butter)
½ teaspoon salt
2 tablespoons chopped, toasted almonds
1 tablespoon raisins
(½ teaspoon cinnamon or ½ teaspoon vanilla or 1 tablespoon lemon juice)

1 recipe Crepe batter

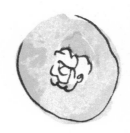

Combine filling ingredients. Preheat oven to 400°F. Prepare the crepes, but do not cook them on their second side. Unlike two-sided crepes, these will stick together if you stack them, so if you don't have a friend working with you, this part takes some space (or else, quite a lot of greased wax paper).

Put 2 big tablespoons of filling on the cooked surface of each crepe. Turn in the sides, and then roll up, making a little golden packet. Place seam-sides down in a well-buttered baking pan and bake for 20 minutes. After the first 10 or 15 minutes, when the bottom is brown, turn to brown the other side. Some filling may escape, but they will be just as good. Blintzes can also be heated on a buttered skillet.

Each filling recipe makes enough for about 12 crepes, which will serve 4, depending.

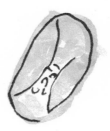

VARIATIONS

More calories

- ↬ Instead of cottage cheese, use ricotta (we freely admit that ricotta is more traditional, in fact).

- ↬ Stir in 2 tablespoons of almond butter into the filling

- ↬ Add an egg yolk to the filling – be sure to cook thoroughly when you include the egg.

- ↬ *Less fat:* Use nonfat cottage cheese and omit butter and nuts.

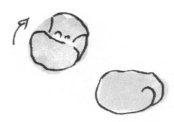

Potatoes!

Have you ever met anyone who wasn't fond of potatoes? The ultimate comfort food. So digestible, and so nutritious, and so *good* – baked, boiled, with butter and parsley, mashed. . . . Here are those essential recipes, for caregivers who didn't learn to cook before 1960.

BAKED

You can bake any potato, but for glorious fluffy insides, choose mature (not "new") potatoes of the "dry" sort, like Idaho or Russet. Cut a thin slice off each end. (That way you can tell if the potato is good; if there's a bad spot it is usually right there to trim out.) Cut a small, deep cross in the center of one of the flatter sides. (That helps prevent the potato from exploding in the oven, which has happened to me – what a mess. The × also makes them easy to "open" at the table.) Put them in a preheated 400°F oven for 40 minutes to an hour, depending on size. Done when a fork pierces easily. You already know about butter and sour cream. I find most yogurt too tart as a nonfat alternative, but buttermilk can be just fine – or non- or low-fat sour cream, or salsa, or . . .

NEW POTATOES

Any potato picked in early summer when it is small and immature counts as "new," but for a real treat, just try the oddball varieties from the farmers market! "Waxy" reds with names like Desirée and Rose Gold, or the golden Butterball, or Yellow Finn, yum. Just scrub them – their skins are thin and tender – and put them in a steamer basket (or boiling water to cover) and cook till tender. The skins of some varieties crack in the prettiest way. Drain, and add a big scoop of chopped parsley while the spuds are still hot enough to cook it. Tiny green peas are lovely too. Butter is traditional, though you can do without it if you need to – easy with Yellow Finns! Salt and pepper. Ah.

Mashed Potatoes

Big mature potatoes are best for mashing (the same kind as for baking). If you get to the farmers market, though, do look for Caribe potatoes, purple-skinned but with creamy-white insides, super for mashing. Or Yukon Gold, so flavorful and buttery-looking that you can skip the butter almost without missing it.

The thing to remember when you make mashed potatoes is keep them *hot* from pot to plate, or else they will set like cement, never to regain their delicacy.

❧

Scrub, trim, and (unless you are an attractive-flecks-of-color fan) peel the potatoes, and cut in quarters. Steam or boil until tender. Some like to include a garlic clove for warmer flavor – cooked this way the taste is not sharp. Drain, and mash with a potato masher or a fork, stirring in the salt and hot milk. Best to serve right away, but if you need to keep them awhile, put their pan into another, larger, pan of hot water, which you can keep simmering gently on the stove.

Leftovers are useful for making soft patties (page 25), for thickening soups, or making Good Shepherd's Pie:

*2 pounds potatoes
  (4-6 potatoes)*
(garlic clove)
1½ teaspoon salt, to taste
*½ cup hot milk, or more, or
  soymilk*

Good Shepherd's Pie is so popular with one vegetarian family we know that they serve it every Thanksgiving, with cranberry sauce and all the other traditional side dishes. It's also an excellent choice for bringing along when you visit someone who is down.

Half fill an 8″ × 8″ pan, or 4 individual pot pie dishes, with lightly cooked mixed vegetables – 4 or 5 cups. Add a cup of flavorful sauce or gravy (or a big onion, sautéed, plus ¾ cup of chopped tomatoes, salt and pepper). Spoon mashed potatoes to cover the top – you will need about a cup, total. A shake of paprika adds color. Bake at 350°F until piping hot, 10 minutes to half an hour – the time will depend on how warm your ingredients were when you started, and the size of the baking dish.

GOOD SHEPHERD'S
PIE

French Bakes

3 large potatoes
1 tablespoon oil
½ teaspoon salt, or to taste
pepper, if desired

A top favorite around our house. They are enough like fries for most of us, with or without ketchup.

Preheat oven to 400°F.

Scrub potatoes and cut into french fry–size pieces. Put them in a bowl with the oil and toss very well, so that each piece is coated with the oil. Spread them on greased cookie sheets one layer deep, and sprinkle with salt. Bake about 35 minutes, or until done to your taste.

Serves 4.

VARIATIONS

With herbs: When tossing with oil, add a handful of favorite herbs, chopped fairly small. We like rosemary, oregano, tarragon.
Shoestrings: Cut potatoes into thin small strips. Spread in one layer on a nonstick pan, and bake until crisp.
Minimum fat: Rinse the potatoes in cold water, and sprinkle with salt before baking. Use much less oil, or none. Bake on a nonstick pan.

GREEN POTATOES
Don't eat green-skinned potatoes, or potato sprouts. Potatoes are a good thing to buy organic, especially in the spring, because of the stuff that's sprayed on non-organic ones to keep them from sprouting.

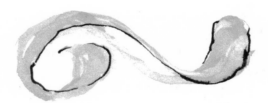

ABOUT PEELS: It used to be almost a matter of religious principle with us that the peels are the best part. Soup, scalloped, mashed, it didn't matter, the peels came along, and we enjoyed every bite. Well, years of gardening and cooking later, we're prepared to admit that once in a while, yes, it's better to peel. A case where that is true is when a patient needs gentle food: the peels are a bit tougher to digest.

To peel, and yet preserve some of the peel nutrients, scrub, trim, quarter, and cook; *then* remove peels.

Potato Soup *Good*

Comforting, digestible, nutritious, easy, and variable, potato soup is a standby, especially for caregivers. Double the amount of base, if you want, so that you can make an entirely different soup later in the week. The base keeps its goodness several days in the refrigerator.

⁘

Wash and trim potatoes, cut in quarters, and steam until tender. Remove from heat and set aside. Meantime, sauté onion and garlic in oil. Slip peels off the potato, unless your eater has the digestive power to manage them.

Mash part or all potato (cube the unmashed part) and stir all of it into the other ingredients. Add liquid as needed. Add salt and pepper.

Add parsley just a few minutes before you serve.

TAILOR THE RECIPE

No fat: Peel potatoes and simmer with garlic and onion in water to cover. Mash or blend, using the water as part of the soup. Good enough for anyone.

More calories: Increase oil for sautéing; use whole milk; stir in sour cream or butter, if the need for calories is very great, and if these improve palatability.

Increase calcium and protein by blending in ½ cup milk powder.

CHOWDER

Potato soup makes a great base for chowder. Add cooked vegetables like these:

- chopped cooked kale (leave some of the potatoes lumpy). + corn — *good*
- tiny green peas (and parsley and potato lumps).
- bits of cooked asparagus, with or without celery and peas.
- chopped, cooked, drained spinach and a little nutmeg.
- corn kernels and a little chopped celery (with leaves).
- mixed cooked vegetables – string beans, carrots, peas, corn…
- lightly cooked broccoli florets and bits of cheddar cheese.
- diced, fresh-cooked artichoke heart, and peas. Add chopped coriander leaves if they are appreciated at your house.

4 large potatoes

1 onion – less

1 2 cloves garlic, or to taste
1 tablespoon olive oil

4 cups hot milk, more or less, or broth or soymilk
1 teaspoon salt, to taste, and pepper
(chopped parsley)

NOTE
Using the blender breaks down the potato's cell structure and that can make gluey soup, particularly if the potato is not cooked thoroughly. Run the blender no longer than necessary. Blending in small batches helps.

Macaroni & Cheese

Sometimes I think we could write a thesis on macaroni and cheese, we have looked at, and tested, so many versions. They have all been good – even the lowest-fat version (6% fat! See margin on next page) was OK if you weren't thinking about what Macaroni & Cheese is like in the Real Fat world.

½ pound macaroni
1–3 cups cream sauce
1–2 cups sharp cheese

Half a pound of macaroni for four people is standard; for that you use a couple of cups of sauce and a cup or so of cheese. Cook macaroni, add cream sauce and cheddar cheese, and, if you have time, bake it, but not longer than what's needed to heat it through.

ADDITIONS

Purists blanch, small children balk. But some others do enjoy the addition of small green peas, sautéed mushrooms, nubbets of asparagus, green beans, broccoli, etc. – even tomato chunks! For a low-fat one-dish meal, add lots of broccoli or asparagus, go easy on sauce, and instead of the cheddar, add (a lot less) Parmesan.

TOPPINGS

A topping of bread crumbs adds appeal. If you bake the macaroni, you don't need to toast the crumbs first, just sprinkle them on. Tossing the crumbs with oil or dotting them with butter makes them crunchier (sigh). Dashes of paprika give color; pepper adds zip.

You can also sprinkle grated cheese on top. Use part of your allotted amount of cheese – the visual impact makes the cheese go farther, and having it on top gives you an easy way to raise or lower the cheese (fat) content of each serving as you spoon it out.

NO DAIRY

Thicken unsweetened grain- or soymilk as suggested in the margin at the top of the next page. If you have not found a nondairy cheddar you like, take a different tack: flavor with sautéed onion, garlic, mushrooms; let a tablespoon of soy sauce or miso stand in for the cheese. Top with crumbs, toasted sesame seeds, chopped nuts.

FLAVOR

Deepen the flavor with onion and garlic. (Turn the page for a recipe!) Some like a dash of red pepper.

Enhance the cheddar taste by adding ½ teaspoon of dry, or 1 teaspoon prepared, mustard.

TAILOR THE RECIPE

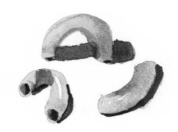

❧ The macaroni: Whole-grain pasta provokes little opposition when used in Mac & Cheese, so here's a fine place to include the flavor, nutrients, and fiber of whole wheat. Try to find whole *durum* wheat macaroni, since that variety of wheat is a golden color, rather than reddish brown. Golden-colored *semolina* isn't whole wheat, it's the refined ("white") flour made from durum wheat. The terminology can get infuriatingly slippery, for sure!

❧ The cheese: Sharp cheddar is standard; milder cheese will give less flavor for the same amount (of cheese, and of fat too).

❧ The sauce: Cream sauce (recipe, pages 34, 42), but you can make it different ways to suit – or use egg instead, see below:
Reduce saturated fat: Use canola or olive oil instead of all or part of the butter. Use reduced-fat cheese; reduce the cheese.
Reduce total fat: For best flavor if you want to lower fat, reduce or eliminate the butter, and keep some cheese.

- ↬ Use much less fat, or none, in the sauce. The trick here is to heat the flour carefully – *avoid browning it* – then add milk gradually, off the heat, stirring like crazy.
- ↬ Use skim milk, or skim milk plus buttermilk for the milk measure. Buttermilk contributes a rich cheesy taste (page 43).

Increase calories

- ↬ When making sauce, add a tablespoon of oil along with butter; use whole milk or whole evaporated milk. Add marble-size pieces of cream cheese to the sauce.
- ↬ Top casserole with oil-toasted crumbs and cheese, wheat germ, chopped nuts. Bake these only briefly, especially the cheese.

For added nutrients

- ↬ Substitute a mixture of egg and milk for the cream sauce (see margin). Bake this version at 325°F until set. The texture will be more custardy than creamy.
- ↬ Blend in ¼ cup milk powder per cup of milk.
- ↬ Top with whole wheat bread crumbs; include wheat germ with the crumbs.

QUICK AND EASY
Effortless creamy sauce:
Cook and drain macaroni
noodles. Put 1 cup in the
blender with hot milk; blend
smooth. Mix into unblended
pasta. Add more milk as
needed, grated cheese, salt,
pepper.

THE 6% SOLUTION
Make the version above with
skim milk and no cheese.
Austere, but not impossible.

½ pound macaroni, cooked
2 or 3 beaten eggs
2 cups warm milk
1 – 2 cups grated cheddar
½ teaspoon salt

Carol's Macaroni & Cheese

Good

1 small onion, chopped
2 cloves garlic
2 tablespoons butter
3 tablespoons flour*
2 cups hot (nonfat) milk
½ teaspoon salt
pepper

½ pound elbow macaroni
   (whole durum flour)
½ pound grated cheddar
   cheese (2 cups)
2 cups whole wheat bread
   crumbs

*(Whole wheat pastry flour
   makes a pale, creamy
   sauce.)*

A primo version that incorporates the added flavor of onion and garlic. The lowered-fat sauce is easier to make because adding the flour to the sautéed onion lets the flour cook without burning, and mix into the milk without lumping. Not exactly a low-fat macaroni, but far less heavy than most, and quite wonderful.

૭

Put a big pot of water on to boil, about 4 quarts, with about ½ tablespoon of salt in it.

Meantime, sauté the onion and garlic in butter, stirring over low heat so that the onion turns golden but does not brown. Crush the garlic with a fork. Add the flour, and stir on low heat for a minute or two, until fragrant; don't let it brown. Add the milk, stirring, and then heat and stir until thick and smooth. Set aside.

When the salted water boils, gradually add the macaroni. Adjust the heat to keep it lively, but not boiling over. When the macaroni is tender – whole wheat pasta takes about 20 minutes – drain it and stir in the sauce and most of the cheese, reserving some for the top. If you like your macaroni soupy, you can add more milk at this point. Adjust salt and pepper.

Put macaroni mixture in a buttered baking dish, and top with the reserved cheese, and bread crumbs. Bake until crumbs are golden brown, about half an hour.

This recipe makes 4 ample, real-world servings. Despite the lowered-fat sauce and moderate cheese, you should know that each serving has 600 calories, 30 grams protein, 26.7 grams fat (40% calories from fat). It is not for every day.

Claudia's Macaroni & Cheese

Delicious and light, with fine flavor. Makes enough to serve your family twice, or to pack half for a friend in need. No one will recognize the buttermilk, it just tastes rich and cheesy.

so

Cook and drain the macaroni, then stir in the buttermilk while the pasta is still hot – it keeps it from sticking together. Also stir in the salt.

Prepare a cream sauce with the oil, flour, and milk. Stir until thick and smooth. Whisk in the mustard, then stir in all but ½ cup of the cheese.

Combine the sauce, and pasta, and correct the salt. If it seems dry at this point you can stir in more milk or buttermilk. Pour in a 9″ × 13″ × 2″ (or 2 8″–square) greased glass baking dish. Top with the remaining cheese. You can add to the topping such things as paprika, whole wheat bread crumbs, wheat germ, more sauce, etc.

Bake at 350°F for half an hour, or until bubbly and golden brown on top.

The recipe makes 10 servings. If you want to compare this recipe with the previous one, each serving has 445 calories, 22 grams protein, 15 grams fat (29% calories from fat).

1½ pounds whole wheat
  macaroni (6 cups)
2 cups buttermilk
2 teaspoons salt, or more

¼ cup oil
¾ cup whole wheat pastry
  flour
5 cups nonfat milk
1 tablespoon prepared
  mustard
  (or 1 teaspoon dry)
2 cups grated cheddar
  cheese

(more milk or buttermilk)

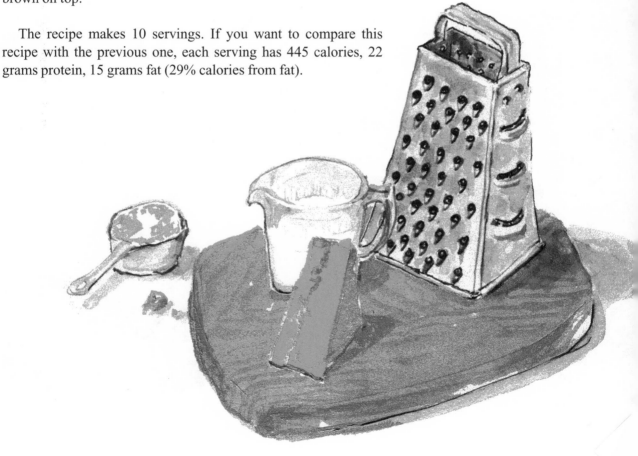

Vegetable Patties . . .

People are fond of patties. Universally appealing on a tender, toasted, wheaty bun, with a fat slice of red ripe tomato, wedge of butter lettuce, pickle, mustard . . . at other times, a patty might surprise you, sitting fragrant and intriguing, there on your plate, when your appetite needs coaxing.

"A great way to get Certain People to eat spinach," says one mom. Certain People opined that leaving out the onion would make it even better.

&

SOFT PATTIES

No need for a rigid recipe here. So easy to put together, we make them all the time, in half a dozen versions.

To make 4, press all the water out of about a cup of cooked spinach, then chop it fine and stir in a bit of sautéed onion and half a cup of ricotta, more or less. Add salt and pepper to taste. Spoon onto bread crumbs on a buttered skillet. When the crumbs are golden, lift the patty with a pancake turner, sprinkle more crumbs on the griddle, turn the patty onto them, and when the second side is golden, you're there. Tender enough for someone who can't chew easily, delectable for anyone. Reduce the fat by using part-skim ricotta, part or all cottage cheese, and a nonstick griddle. Serve plain, or with chutney or salsa, or in the middle of a spot of smoothly puréed red or yellow bell pepper . . .

Instead of spinach: Swiss chard. Grilled red bell pepper. Grated or thin-sliced asparagus (add Parmesan). Artichoke heart (& leaf-scrapings – sauté garlic with the onion; add Parmesan cheese, and a few green peas; plenty of pepper). If the mixture tastes good to you before you cook it, it will make a nice patty.

These are very soft and tender, not bunnable.

For potato patties, turn to page 25.

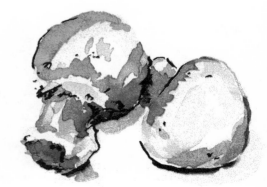

. . . & Burgers

🍂 Grate a big zucchini and toss with half a teaspoon of salt. Let it drain in a colander for an hour, then mix with lots of parsley, bread crumbs, grated cheese, and an egg. Cook until tender.

🍂 Chop 2 cups of mushroom pieces fine. Add to sautéing onion and garlic, and cook until their color changes. Add ½ cup cooked grated potato, or rice, or other cooked grain. Salt and pepper, soy sauce, a handful of cheese, if wanted. (You can add 1 or 2 beaten eggs after the mixture cools slightly. This will make patties hold together firmly.) Cook on crumbs or sesame seeds. Good in buns.

✧ Bake formed, breaded patties on a cookie sheet. Turn once.

✧ Fast and easy: spread mixture to fill a greased baking sheet. Bake, cut, then lift with spatula – works fine, even on buns.

✧ Easy veggie "burgers" to *grill:* Marinate round, 1″-thick slices of a big eggplant in soy sauce or barbecue sauce. Grill, and make your burger around it. Yum. Juicy and savory.

✧ A favorite with our teenagers: Ready-made tempeh patties.

Walnut Oatmeal Burgers

The best. Grind walnuts in blender or processor, and combine with oats, eggs, milk, onion, sage, salt, and pepper. If you are using a processor, remove the nuts, chop the onions, then combine everything. Form into patties.

Brown 5 on both sides on a lightly oiled skillet (or 10 on 2 skillets), then pour in the stock, and bring to a boil. Reduce heat to low, cover, and simmer 25 minutes. Serve on buns with "the fixin's," or crumble, and use instead of hamburger in chili beans, spaghetti sauce, etc.

Makes about 10 burgers, rather a lot. Rather than halve the amount, why not cook half and freeze the rest to cook at another time? – or else, while munching on the first, simmer the second batch, then freeze them to star another day. Sturdy enough to reheat on the barbecue grill.

Half a cup of partly-cooked, grated potato will hold patties together almost as well as an egg. Press them firmly to shape.

A reminder: if you add egg, taste before the egg goes in.

ALTERNATE ROUTES
FOR COOKING

ALTERNATE
BURGERS

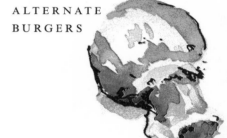

1½ – 3 cups walnut pieces
2 cups rolled oats
3 or 4 eggs, slightly beaten
½ cup skim milk
1 large onion, chopped fine
1 teaspoon sage
1 teaspoon salt
freshly ground black pepper
    to taste
oil to brown patties
3 cups vegetable stock

A Few Sweet Things

Caring and sweetness express themselves *a lot* of ways besides "somethin' from the oven." Even so, sweets will always have their place in the scheme of things. There's some old, deep wisdom in the belief that when you, with loving heart, prepare and give a delectable sweet treat, you may for a short time ease the bitterness of someone's sickness, or even, their sadness. When someone's having a rough time, getting a moment of distraction from the pain and routine *can* sometimes help reset their mental picture, make everything seem a little more hopeful.

Obviously, we are not talking about loading up on fat and sugar *often*. That's a bad idea, and an especially bad idea for a sick body struggling to get well. You as cook exercise your discrimination and artistry in this. But custards, puddings, fruit concoctions, even ice cream from the market! – such as these can provide needed nourishment at times to someone who otherwise wouldn't be able to handle it.

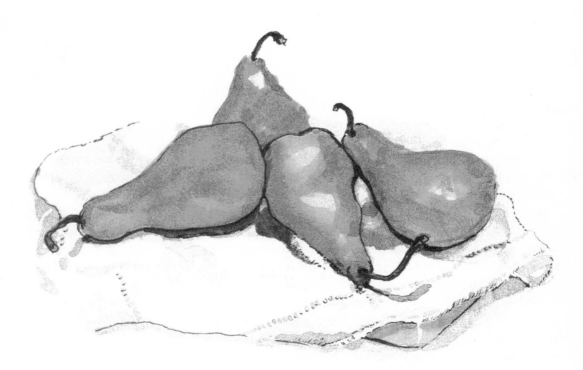

Baked Apples

Baked apples surprise you with how good they are, all by themselves or with yogurt or, need I add, with vanilla ice cream. Most kinds of apples work well enough, except the "Delicious" varieties, especially Yellow Delicious, which stay firm no matter how long you bake them.

You don't *need* a recipe. Just find a deep baking dish with a good lid. Put apples in it until they fit snugly, then take them out again and core them, and put them back right-side-up. If there are spaces, halve or quarter another apple or two, and stick them around the holes. Fill the centers of the whole apples with granola, or with the indicated mixture. If the apples are very tart, add extra sugar. Pour an inch of apple juice (or water) around the apples and bake, tightly covered, until they are soft. Four normal apples take about 40 minutes at 350°F.

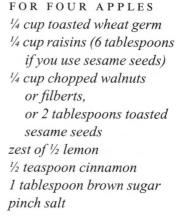

FOR FOUR APPLES
¼ cup toasted wheat germ
¼ cup raisins (6 tablespoons if you use sesame seeds)
¼ cup chopped walnuts or filberts, or 2 tablespoons toasted sesame seeds
zest of ½ lemon
½ teaspoon cinnamon
1 tablespoon brown sugar
pinch salt

See pages 88–89 for Applesauce and Stewed Apples.

Tapioca "Gell-O"

Here is a gelled dessert entirely for fun. Very pretty, with a mellow, rich flavor that's entirely superior to any other version of gelled dessert we have met. If your patient's digestion is not robust, substitute soft, less acidic fruits. See pages 90, 91, and 132 for other recipes and suggestions.

Mix everything and let stand 5 minutes. Bring *just* to the boiling point, then immediately remove from heat. Stir a few times while it cools.

Makes 2½ delicious cups – very like jello except instead of smoothly clear it is attractively rippley.

2 cups sweet red fruit juice
3 tablespoons instant tapioca
¼ cup dried cranberries
¼ cup diced soft dried apricots

UNCLEAR!
Please note that unlike animal gelatin or agar, tapioca qualifies for a "full liquid" but not "clear liquid" diet.

Vanilla Pudding

4 cups fresh milk
¼ cup cornstarch
½ cup brown sugar
¼ teaspoon salt
1–2 teaspoons vanilla

To prevent a skin from forming on the top, stir pudding once or twice as it cools.

PLEASE NOTE:
Some good cooks maintain that cornstarch tastes raw unless it has cooked fully 10 minutes. See what you think. For such longer cooking, make the pudding in a double boiler.

A stainless steel bowl that fits snugly on top of your saucepan and hangs an inch above the level of simmering water makes a working double boiler.

To some of us, vanilla pudding is the ultimate comfort food, quick and easy to make from on-hand staples. Adaptable to suit widely differing needs and tastes.

Measure the milk and pour all but about ½ cup of it into a heavy saucepan. Heat, stirring often enough to prevent the milk from scorching – the less fat the milk has, the more careful you need to be. As the milk in the pan nears boiling, stir the cornstarch into the ½ cup reserved milk, dissolving the starch completely. Add a little of the hot milk to that, mixing them together; pour warm cornstarch mixture into hot milk, stirring gently until the mixture comes to a boil and thickens somewhat. Remove from heat.* Add the sugar and salt, stirring, still gently, until they are dissolved. Cool a bit, then stir in the vanilla.

Serve warm or cold.

Pudding thickens much more as it cools. Keeps several days in the refrigerator – cover the container to protect flavor.

Recipe makes 8 half-cup servings, or 4 one-cup servings. Very good plain or topped with berries or other sweet or stewed fruit, or anything you'd put on ice cream.

TAILOR THE RECIPE

↬ *To add the nutrients of egg:* Prepare as directed, up to taking the pan off the fire. Stir half a cup of the hot pudding into one or two beaten eggs, then strain that into the main pudding. Return the pot to low heat and let it just come to the boil, stirring gently, then take it off the fire.

↬ *No fat:* Tastes surprisingly good made with skim milk if you are on a no-fat regime. When skim milk gets close to boiling, it can foam up, so choose a pan big enough to hold twice the quantity. Measure everything out ahead of time so that you can stir continuously to prevent scorching. If you fix this often, a double boiler will make life a lot easier.

For Cup Custard, see page 129.

Classic Rice Pudding

Worth eating, even when nothing else seems to be. The brown rice makes the dish more nutritious, and won't be noticed if the rice is cooked soft.

Preheat oven to 325°F. Combine ingredients and pour into a greased baking dish. Dot with butter if desired, and a dash of cinnamon or nutmeg. Bake until set, about half an hour – more if your ingredients started out cold.

Serves 6 generously.

2 cups well-cooked brown
    rice
2 cups milk
½ cup brown sugar
1 teaspoon vanilla
2 eggs
(zest of a lemon)
(½ cup raisins)

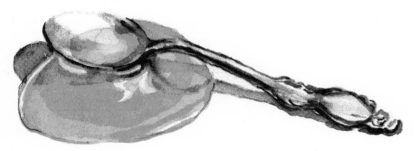

Easy Spooning Rice Pudding

Quick and satisfying, and a very flexible recipe.

Mix rice and milk in double boiler and heat slowly on a back burner until rice is very soft. Blend ⅔ cup of the mixture smooth in blender and return it to the pan. Remove from heat and sweeten to taste. Serve plain or add a dash of cinnamon, or the zest of a lemon. Good with fresh berries or stewed fruit.

2 cups well-cooked brown
    rice, more or less
2 cups milk or soymilk, more
    or less
¼ cup brown sugar or honey,
    or other sweetener, to
    taste

VARIATIONS

↪ *Khir:* Add ¼ teaspoon of crushed cardamom seeds. Skip the cinnamon.

↪ *Smooth and creamy rice pudding:* Blend all of the pudding smooth in the blender, adjusting thickness with extra milk if needed.

↪ *Nuggety:* Add diced dried fruit and nuts.

Bread Pudding

4 slices of airy whole wheat
  bread, lightly buttered
2 cups warm milk
2 eggs, slightly beaten
⅓ cup brown sugar, or other
  sweetener

Preheat oven to 325°F.

Cut the bread into cubes and put in a greased 8″ × 8″ pan. Mix the rest of the ingredients and pour over the bread. Bake about 45 minutes – done when delicately brown on top. Let stand 5 to 10 minutes before serving.

VARIATIONS

↬ *For added flavor:* Add a teaspoon of vanilla. Lemon zest. Cinnamon.

↬ *For added protein:* Add half a cup cottage cheese.

↬ *For added calories:* Use whole milk; dot top with butter and sprinkle with sugar and cinnamon. Add ½ cup cut dried fruit, raisins, nuts, etc.

৯৹

Savory Bread Pudding: Need not butter the bread. Substitute grated swiss or sharp cheddar cheese for the sweetener. Can add sautéed onion, garlic, celery, grilled bell peppers. Serve with a pile of dark green vegetables, plus fresh tomato salad, or salsa, or chutney alongside.

Gingerbread

This simplified recipe is splendid, and all possible variations have been enthusiastically received. It is amazingly good. The whole wheat flour will not be detected even by those who otherwise resist healthy food.

⅓ cup oil
1 cup molasses
1⅓ cups buttermilk

2½ cups whole wheat flour
1 teaspoon soda
1 teaspoon cinnamon
2 teaspoons ground ginger
½ teaspoon salt
(¼ – ½ teaspoon powdered mustard)
(½ cup raisins)

ॐ

Preheat oven to 350°F. Grease an 8″ or 9″ square pan.

Mix oil, molasses, and buttermilk.

Sift dry ingredients together and combine with the wets. Add raisins if wanted.

Turn into greased pan and bake about 45 minutes – a bit longer for 8″, a bit less for 9″.

Let cool in pan at least 10 minutes.

Serves 6 generously, 9 with ice cream. Just as good with yogurt. Makes great muffins too – bake them about 25 minutes.

TAILORING THE RECIPE

↬ *To add the nutrients of egg:* Substitute an egg for ¼ cup of the buttermilk. Milder flavor, lighter texture.

↬ *No fat:* Substitute prune purée for the oil. Cook an extra 10 minutes. Flavor is excellent, mysteriously fruity. Texture is moister. This version adds fiber and iron. (Prune purée: pit 3 medium raw or stewed prunes, and blend smooth with their own liquid, or water, to cover. If you have the small cup-size blender jar, use that.) Some testers like this version best of all.

↬ *No dairy:* Substitute orange juice for buttermilk. A lot of our friends say *this* version is the very best. Can add some grated orange peel, too, if wanted. The orange juice version made fat-free with prune purée rated high with our testers.

↬ *Fancy:* Add minced crystallized ginger.

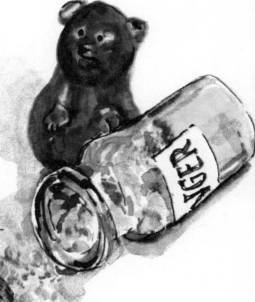

Glena's Pumpkin Pie

2 cups cooked pumpkin or
winter squash
or 1 pound pumpkin
(small can)
½ cup honey (or brown
sugar)
2 eggs (scant half cup)
½ teaspoon salt
1 – 1½ teaspoons cinnamon
½ –1 teaspoon ginger
⅛ teaspoon cloves
1 can (13 oz.) evaporated
milk

For a home-pantry version
of evaporated milk, blend
⅓ cup milk powder with
1⅓ cups milk

For almost everyone, pumpkin pie evokes fragrant memories of warm family times and simple joys. That makes it a fine choice to take to anyone who needs cheering up. Our dear friend Glena Records goes to visit cancer patients, and she likes to take along this pie, made from her homegrown pumpkin. It provides substantial nutrition along with the dose of nostalgia. In addition, the pumpkin is easy to eat, and easy to keep down, even for people with stomachs shaky from medication, chemotherapy, radiation – or for any number of reasons.

Mix smooth. Pour into unbaked fluted pie shell. Bake at 425°F for 15 minutes, then lower heat to 350°F and bake another 45 minutes.

TAILORING THE RECIPE

↪ *Lower the fat:* Use evaporated skim milk. Substitute 4 egg whites, or nonfat egg replacer, for the eggs. Cook the filling in a greased glass pie pan, without the crust.

↪ *More calories:* Increase the eggs to 3. Use whole evaporated milk.

↪ *More protein:* Increase eggs to 3. Blend an extra ⅓ cup milk powder into the milk.

↪ *For easy spoon-feeding* (and gentler digesting): Cook the filling in custard cups instead of the pie shape. For best texture, place the filled cups in a pan of hot water while baking. (See pages 124–125 for baking tips.)

↪ *No dairy:* Omit milk and egg. Increase pumpkin to 4 cups. Start with smaller amount of seasoning, and adjust to taste.

Friend to Friend

"Breakfast can be an act of caring," says a writer who gives time-saving ideas in the Wednesday Food Page. This week she proposes "a gift for a friend in need" – a breakfast casserole to assemble by layering the contents of four cans and a couple of plastic pouches from the supermarket freezer case. The writer says, "They can heat it when they want it."

This scenario didn't appeal much to me – all that plastic, and not even cooked! Margarita, who is a nurse, was looking over my shoulder. She said softly, "How very thoughtful it is to take a casserole to someone who is having a rough time." That stopped me, and I had to admit, gee, even such a simple offering probably would be awfully welcome. I mean, sure, it'd be great if you made lasagna with homemade noodles and just-picked garden spinach. But – splendid as the grand gesture definitely *is* – something nutritious and easy, even something very simple, might be just as much help and mean just as much. If the rough time might go on for a while, that gift casserole can be particularly welcome a little later, after the newness of the situation has passed, and the caregiving is settling into a routine that may begin to seem pretty bleak.

Another sort of gift to bring is an afternoon's respite – take the caregiver for a walk on the beach, or shopping – or to a show, where their mind will be diverted and refreshed. If they cannot arrange to leave for an afternoon, think of bringing some amusement, not the least of which would be your own funny stories and anecdotes.

Almost anything from "Comfort Foods" would be a great choice for taking to a friend. Collected in the next few pages, though, you'll find some of our particular favorites for this purpose, recipes perfect for packing, or especially tailored for the needs of caregivers; for example, many of us have had the experience of putting on weight when we were looking after a very ill family member. It isn't only the inactivity. Anxiety, grief, frustration can send almost anyone seeking chocolate. You've got to have a break from the tension and worry. You only have one minute. A chocolate truffle is so intense, and so quick! Total escape in a plumb bob. No one claims they're good for the

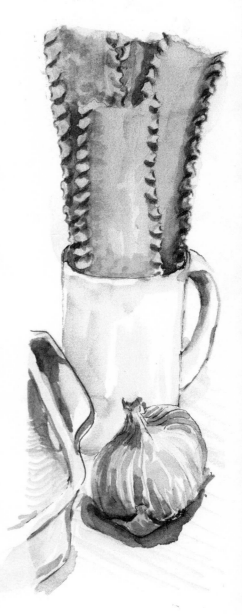

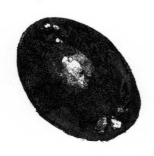

body . . . If you know someone who's in this situation, try to supply some delectable munchies that are low fat, low calorie, and healthful, to help them keep the number of plumb bobs down, and their long-term health up. My particular fad is perfectly ripe, organic whole kumquats, in season. Somewhat more universal would be . . .

Caregivers' Brownies

1 cup prune purée*
1½ cups sugar
1 egg white, lightly beaten
1½ teaspoons vanilla

1 cup unsweetened
   cocoa powder
1¼ cups whole wheat flour
   or oat flour
1½ teaspoons baking
   powder
¼ teaspoon salt

A bittersweet chocolate hit, very intense. As written, it has no added fat at all and is dense and fudgy-chewy. There are plenty of ways to vary it, however – some suggested below.

Why the prune purée? Prunes contain sorbitol, a form of sugar that holds moisture; they also have a lot of pectin, which makes them hold air bubbles somewhat. These enable them to behave effectively as a substitute, in equal measure, for fat in some kinds of baked goods – and this is one.

જ

Preheat oven to 350°F. Grease a 9″ x 13″ pan.

Mix liquids and sugar. Sift dry ingredients separately, then combine them with the wets in a big bowl. Pour into the baking dish, spreading the top flat with a knife or spatula.

Bake about 20 to 25 minutes. It's done when it shrinks from sides of pan, and the center springs back to a light touch. Cool at least 10 minutes before cutting. Store extras in the refrigerator.

TAILORING THE RECIPE

Add orange zest (grated peel) or, if fat is not a crucial issue, chopped walnuts, pecans, even chocolate chips.

For a cakier version, still moist, however: Substitute 1 or 2 eggs or 4 egg whites for an equal amount of the purée, and add ½ teaspoon more baking soda to the dry ingredients.

For a fancier presentation: Before cutting, spread baked, partly cooled brownies with seedless raspberry jam and a dusting of powdered sugar or sliced almonds.

*PRUNE PURÉE
Put about 12 large prunes (⅓ pound) in water to cover, and simmer until soft. Cool, remove the pits, and blend with the juice that remained in the pan. You can also blend or process a cup of uncooked chopped pitted prunes with ½ cup water. (Quantities here are flexible. In our many tests, nothing didn't work.)

Lasagna al Forno

Perhaps the top favorite of all casseroles. This version is almost complete nutritionally, with a reasonably low fat level, making it ideal for bringing to a "friend in need."

> ❧

Cook noodles in a very large shallow pan of boiling, salted water until *almost* tender; they will cook more in the oven, absorbing liquid from the sauce as they do, and if they are still firm at this point, they'll hold together better while you're assembling the dish. After draining the noodles, it can be helpful to spread them out on a towel or waxed paper, or submerge them in cold water.

Grease a 9″ x 13″ x 2½″ baking dish, or two 8″ x 8″ pans. Spread a thin layer of sauce in the bottom, and then a layer of noodles, lengthwise. Keep the best of the noodles for the top and use broken ones in the middle. Each layer of noodles should lie crosswise to the one below it.

On the layer of noodles, spread the first layer of filling: ½ the cottage cheese, ⅓ of the nuts, ¼ of the Parmesan; then a coating of sauce. Layer noodles again, then the spinach and most of the mozzarella, and sauce. More noodles, another cheese and nuts layer, and your prettiest noodles across the top. Add sauce and the rest of the nuts and cheese for the top.

Bake covered at 350°F for 30 to 45 minutes (if your ingredients were hot, the shorter time will be enough). Uncover for the last 10 minutes. Let stand another 10 minutes before cutting – otherwise it will be too runny to hold together, and too hot to eat.

Serves 8.

TAILORING THE RECIPE

Faster preparation: If you can allow a longer baking time, you do not have to cook the noodles beforehand. Cover the casserole tightly while baking about an hour.

No dairy: Use soy cheeses, or substitute grated tofu for the mozzarella and omit the other cheeses. For good results with this version, your sauce should be very flavorful.

¾ *pound whole wheat or whole wheat-soy lasagna noodles*
6 *cups tomato sauce*

2 *cups cottage cheese*
3 *cups grated mozzarella or Swiss cheese (10 oz.)*
1–3 *bunches spinach**
½ *cup grated Parmesan cheese*
¾ *cup chopped toasted walnuts or almonds*

*The spinach can be either raw or cooked. If raw, 1 large bunch will be enough: wash, shake dry, and chop fine. Cooking ahead lets you use more spinach – 3 big bunches or even more. Cook with only the water that clings to the leaves, drain well; chop fine.

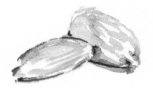

Minestrone

1 onion, chopped
2 cloves garlic
1½ cups chopped celery
1½ tablespoons olive oil
4 cups chopped tomatoes,
  with juice, fresh or
  canned
2 bay leaves
1 teaspoon oregano
2 teaspoons basil
pinch fennel seed

2 cups or more bite-size,
  cooked vegetables:
  carrot, zucchini, potato,
  broccoli, green beans,
  peas, corn, green pepper,
  cabbage, sautéed
  mushrooms

1 cup cooked beans: lima,
  kidney, pinto, black,
  garbanzo

handful of raw or cooked
  whole wheat pasta

(½ cup cooked grain)
salt to taste
plenty of pepper

(tender greens, cut up)
½ cup chopped parsley

Minestrone is easy to prepare, and a universal favorite. A good choice to take to a snuffly friend, or to a caregiving one. The recipe makes enough for them, and for your family too. A bowl of minestrone alongside a good green salad and crusty bread, with juicy pears for dessert – what could be better?

⁂

Begin with the tomato soup base and include your choice of grains, beans, and vegetables.

Sauté onion, garlic, and celery in oil until soft. Crush garlic. Add tomatoes and herbs. Simmer this base gently while you prepare whatever vegetables, beans, or grains you wish to add.

Add beans, noodles, and/or the grain half an hour before you want to serve the soup, so the flavors can marry.

Minestrone welcomes leftover cooked vegetables. If you are preparing fresh, steam or simmer them separately before adding to the soup – vegetables cooked in tomato lose their color. Add vegetable cooking water to the soup. Parsley and tender greens will keep their color and not overcook if you add them just a few minutes before serving. Don't count them as part of the 2 cups of vegetables because they cook down so much; just add them as extras.

After combining all the ingredients, bring the soup to a boil, simmer briefly, and check the salt. If you like, garnish each bowl with a spoonful of Parmesan cheese.

Makes about 10 cups – all to the good because it's even better the next day.

Serves 6 generously.

Enchiladas Petaluma

This recipe is rather fabulous as written – including how long it takes to prepare. But the quick and easy version is plenty good: use corn tortillas, diced leftover vegetables, and a prepared sauce.

One day, though, do the whole thing from scratch – you won't believe how good it is.

If you are making your own crepes, blend the ingredients briefly and set aside. If using the fresh corn and/or onion mixture, blend that first with the milk until it is smooth, then blend briefly with the other ingredients. Prepare the vegetables and sauce. Make the crepes, adding more liquid as needed to adjust the batter so it will make a thin crepe. (See page 32 for crepe-making instructions.)
If you are using tortillas, soften each one by warming it on burner or griddle, then brush lightly with oil before filling.
To make sauce, sauté the onion and garlic in oil in a big skillet, adding the cumin and chili when the onion is translucent; cook gently until golden. Crush the garlic with a fork. Add the tomatoes and salt, and cook until softened. If tomatoes are watery, cook off most of the water.

Mix the vegetables with half the sauce and most of the cilantro. Fill each crepe or tortilla with about ⅓ cup of the mixture, placing them in two rows, seam down, in a 9″ x 13″ pan (or fill 2 8″ square pans). Top with remaining sauce. Cover and bake 20 minutes at 350°F, or a bit longer if the vegetables were cold. Sprinkle with more cheese, if you want, and the rest of the cilantro.

Serves 2, 3, or 4, depending.

8 Corn Crepes or tortillas
Vegetable Mixture
2 cups Mexican Sauce
2 bunches cilantro leaves,
   chopped

CORN CREPES
½ cup cornmeal; or fresh-
   cooked corn off 1 cob
1 cup milk or water
½ cup whole wheat flour
2 eggs or 4 whites
½ teaspoon salt
(½ minced sautéed onion &
   garlic, ½ teaspoon cumin
   added and cooked in)

SAUCE
a big onion, chopped fine
5 cloves garlic
2 tablespoons oil
1 tablespoon ground cumin
(2 green chilis, chopped fine,
   or hot pepper to taste)
3 cups red ripe tomatoes,
   peeled, seeded, chopped
1 teaspoon salt, to taste

VEGETABLE MIX
2 each, grilled green, red,
   yellow peppers, diced
¾ cup cooked, drained,
   chopped spinach
(½ cup each, grated jack and
   cheddar cheese)
¼ cup sliced black olives
salt and pepper to taste

Green Rice Casserole

*1 small bunch scallions
or an onion
1 small clove garlic
oil for sautéing
2½ cups cooked brown rice
⅓ cup chopped parsley
½ cup grated swiss cheese
2 eggs, lightly beaten
2 cups milk
¾ – 1 teaspoon salt*

Intensely nutritious, Green Rice Casserole is just the thing to tempt the appetite of someone who needs that, and so, a prime candidate for carrying to the hospital or home when a friend is convalescing. If you are taking it to a caregiver, maybe bring along ripe tomatoes and greens for salad as well.

Preheat oven to 350°F.

Chop scallions or onion and sauté with garlic in oil until soft. Crush the garlic with a fork. Combine with rest of the ingredients, using the smaller amount of salt if the rice was already salted. Pour the mixture into a greased 2-quart casserole. Bake about 45 minutes, until set. Cool slightly if you want to cut it in tidy squares.

TAILOR THE RECIPE

↪ *Lower fat:* Cut the cheese in half and use skim milk. Substitute 4 egg whites for the whole eggs.

↪ *No dairy:* Omit the cheese, milk, and eggs. Add plenty of sautéed mushrooms, and chopped grilled bell peppers. A very different dish, lighter – delicious.

↪ *Bland, but good:* Leave out the sautéed onion and garlic.

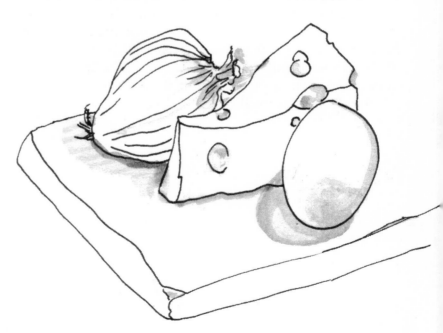

Diana's Baked Vegetables

Very easy to do, and a long-standing favorite. The recipe is large because our testers liked the leftovers so much. Some ideas they offered for using them are given below. You can also divide the ingredients into two, to use one at home and gift the other.

Alternative vegetables that work: green beans, winter squash, brussels sprouts, carrots. Leeks instead of onions. In winter, omit the tomato and use turnips, carrots, beets, potatoes. Aim for balance in the flavors if you choose different veggies.

᠗

Preheat oven to 350°F.

Scrub, trim, and cut vegetables into bite-size pieces – potatoes smallest. Mix the second group of ingredients in a large bowl, then add the vegetables and stir to be sure all are coated with sauce.

Grease a deep 9″ x 13″ baking dish, or 2 8″ x 8″ dishes, and transfer the mixture into it or them. Cover tightly. Bake for an hour. Vegetables should be tender, most of the sauce absorbed. If they look soupy, stir them and return uncovered to oven for 10 or 15 minutes. This is important, because it intensifies the flavor and "makes" the dish.

Six generous servings. Goes very well over brown rice. Since there is not much *green* here, we suggest serving with a spinach or mixed green salad.

TESTERS SUGGEST

↝ Great the next day for lunch.

↝ Toss the leftovers with cooked pasta and serve hot; or cold, for a delicious pasta salad. If you plan ahead for this, you can make this half of the vegetables without potato.

↝ Makes a great vegetable layer in lasagna.

↝ Add to Golden Broth or one of the Tomato Soups to make a hearty, stewey soup.

↝ For a more "roasted" effect, use two big flat pans and cook *uncovered* at 450°F for only half an hour.

1 potato
1 medium eggplant
2 or 3 zucchini or other
  summer squashes
2 or 3 red, yellow, &/or
  green bell peppers
(1– 3 cups mushrooms)

2½ cups peeled tomatoes,
  fresh or canned
1 onion, chopped big
3 cloves garlic, quartered
¼ cup olive oil
1 teaspoon salt
plenty of pepper

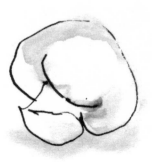

Fruit Salad

oranges, grapefruit,
    tangerines
peaches, nectarines,
    mangoes, papaya
pineapple

berries: strawberries,
    blueberries,
    brambleberries . . .
grapes

melon balls

Once in a while,
    a few lightly toasted
    almonds, cashews,
    pecans, sometimes
    walnuts, pistachios

lightly toasted coconut

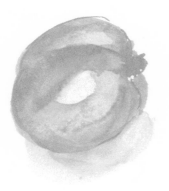

There just is nothing better than a good fruit salad. Think of taking one to a friend who's down – what could possibly be more welcome? So delightful, so pretty, fresh, and health giving.

The basic great fruit salad consists of ripe, but not overripe, bananas cut in half lengthwise, then in ¼″ slices, plus oranges, peeled with a knife and cut into slightly larger chunks. Toss together long enough to coat the banana with orange juice, which keeps it from getting brown. For dressy occasions, once in a while add lightly toasted coconut to make Ambrosia. But go easy on the coconut, here and in general, please.

In winter, add chunks of meltingly ripe pear; or grapefruit and tangerine sections. Winter oranges with tough membranes, and grapefruits, do well to have their membranes removed. This is not hard to do, though it does take a little bit of time. Peel the fruit with a sharp knife, removing the outside membrane with the peel. Then cut toward the center of the fruit along each membrane, pulling the sections free from the "core". Grapefruit prepared in this way makes a wonderful addition to fruit salad because it has just enough bitterness to provide counterpoint to the sweetness of the other winter fruits.

For added color, a few pomegranate dots, or slices of kiwi. Once in a while, the really gooey-sweet dates that are available in winter are good cut up in these salads. Mostly, dried fruit is too chewy and too intense.

In summer, you may want to leave out the citrus to showcase ripe peaches and the other glorious summer fruits. Usually you do want to keep some banana, unless there are ripe figs. A very sweet offering. Grapes are good if they are quite small. Otherwise, halve them. A bit of something slightly tart can be an improvement – berries, a little squeeze of lemon, even small amounts of relatively sweet plums, cut thin, can sometimes work. If you use tender raspberries, olallies, boysenberries, etc., add them at the last minute, folding them gently into the mixture so they don't fall apart or (worse) discolor the whole thing. The softest berries, just strew on top. Hard, sour plums and apricots spell ruin.

Melons often find their way into fruit salad. Sometimes they can be all right, especially if they are made into balls with a melon baller. But melon has a different ambiance, so be cautious. Bananas and melons usually fight, for example. And the happy eater who bites into cantaloupe whilst expecting peach or mango cannot but be disappointed, no matter how good the cantaloupe.

The primo way to use melons is in an all-melon-ball combo like honeydew, Crane, and Charlaine, or even honeydew, watermelon, and cantaloupe, and stop there. Melons should be perfectly ripe, but if they need a little help, dissolve a spoonful of sugar in the juice of a lemon, and lace it on. Serve in wine glasses garnished with a sprig of mint – very pretty, very refreshing on a hot day.

Ripe pineapple works with almost anything (except melon). Do be sure to remove all the little prickly stickers.

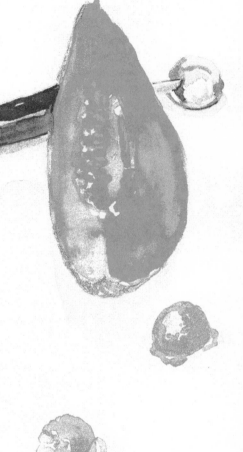

BASIC PRINCIPLES

- Avoid using the thin-bladed carbon-steel knives. Their high iron content gives acid fruit a metallic taste.

- The larger the number of kinds of fruit, the more careful you have to be that they work well together. Always consider color.

- Hardly ever do you need to add sweetener. Even if the first bite seems a tiny bit tart, the second will taste just right, and the salad will be so much more refreshing than it would if it were loaded down with sugar. Honey, as a rule, has such a powerful presence that you can scarcely taste the fruit. Occasionally a dab of marmalade will save the day, however.

- *Please don't include hard pears, or apples.* They strike a disharmonious textural note when combined with soft fruits. Elsewhere, apples shine in so many outstanding dishes – Waldorf salad with celery, walnuts, and a creamy dressing. Grated into carrot salad or cole slaw. Baked. And, ah yes, Apple Crisp . . .

Apple Crisp

8 apples
juice of 1 lemon
1 teaspoon cinnamon
2 tablespoons whole wheat
  flour
¾ cup raisins
water or apple juice

TOPPING

1 cup rolled oats
⅓ cup toasted wheat germ
½ cup whole wheat flour
½ teaspoon salt
2 teaspoons cinnamon
½ cup brown sugar
½ cup butter (or oil)

Good

Many friends declare that this homey confection is The Very Best Dessert, better than pie. Easier than pie, too. Great the next day, too, so it is a primo choice for taking to a friend.

❧

Preheat oven to 375°F. Peel and slice apples until you have enough to fill a greased 9″ × 13″ baking dish, or two 8″ × 8″ dishes. Mix the apples with lemon juice, cinnamon, flour, and raisins in a bowl, then transfer them to the baking dish, adding enough water or apple juice to cover the bottom. Water is fine unless the apples don't have much flavor.

Mix topping in a bowl and press onto top of apples. Bake uncovered for 25 minutes, or until the apples are soft.

Serves 8.

OBSERVATIONS

Any kind of apple works, but green pippins and others with a lot of tart flavor are fabulous. Sweet apples like Gravensteins at their peak may permit a reduction of sugar. Contemplate Yellow Delicious reluctantly. They don't soften.

Fruits other than apples can be outrageously delicious in this recipe. We have had success with winter pears, peaches, apricots. (Unless apricots are supersweet and ripe, sweeten the fruit to taste in addition to the measure of sugar in the topping.) And plums (ditto on the sugar). The recipe is a champ at transforming otherwise unglamorous or oversupplied stuff into a celebration.

The "serve with" list starts with yogurt and goes along through ice cream and vanilla pudding, and their nondairy analogs – you know, all the usual suspects. Excellent plain, also.

Plenty of Fluids

"Get some rest and drink plenty of fluids, and you'll feel better in a few days." Did you ever wonder *why* it works?

WHY EMPHASIZE DRINKING FLUIDS FOR A COLD OR FLU?

❧ Hot liquids, especially aromatic herbal teas and broths, work immediately to clear sinuses. When there is fever, hot liquids encourage sweating, helping to cool the body without interfering with the fever's germ-fighting work.

❧ When you have a cold, drinking plenty of fluid dilutes mucus, so it can drain. That relieves sinus pressure, and you feel better right away. Also, mucus that is diluted is less likely to become infected than if it is thick and sticky.

❧ Liquids soothe a scratchy throat, and keep postnasal drainage from making a sore throat worse.

❧ The body loses vital fluid and electrolytes even from a runny nose, or sweating from fever. Diarrhea and vomiting cause much greater losses. Replacing lost fluid protects against dehydration, especially urgent for babies, for older patients, for anyone who is not robust. Dehydration is extremely serious, and requires immediate medical attention. Prevention is better.home-brew salts

REHYDRATION

News reports tell dramatic stories about the UN volunteers using oral rehydration salts to miraculously save the lives of poor children in countries across the globe. American babies sometimes get diarrhea too. Every mother should know that the neighborhood pharmacy carries oral rehydration packets! It is a good idea to keep some in your medicine cabinet. They can save a child's life.

For sickies who are over 12:
1 quart water
½ teaspoon baking soda
½ teaspoon table salt
3 tablespoons sugar
1 teaspoon salt substitute, if available ("lite salt")

WHAT IS "PLENTY" OF FLUIDS?

❧ Aim for a cup of liquid every waking hour for a grown-up who has a cold or flu – half that for a child of 100 pounds, etc.

❧ Check urine color: if it's clear, pale yellow, fluid intake is OK.

❧ *Caregivers! Protect your own health by doing the same – and wash your hands often. Keep hands away from your nose and eyes, which are even more susceptible to contagion than your mouth. Get plenty of sleep if you possibly can, and walks in the sunshine.*

WHAT DO THEY MEAN BY "CLEAR" LIQUIDS?

❧ The test is, if you put it in a glass, you can see your hand through the glass. Water, weak black tea, weak herbal teas like camomile or raspberry leaf; mild clear broth, diluted apple juice. Avoid acidic beverages unless they are diluted. Warm is better than cold.

❧ Whey is a clear liquid for most purposes, and the only good-quality protein source in this category. (Animal gelatin, normally considered a clear liquid, is protein, but extremely poor quality.)

Whey powder is sometimes available; check the ingredient list to make sure there's nothing "unclear" added.

You can make your own whey, though as a protein source it would be dilute, only 1.9 grams per cup. Put a quart of mild-tasting nonfat yogurt in a coffee filter (or in a finely woven cloth napkin set in a colander) and let it stand undisturbed in the refrigerator for several hours or longer. The whey will drip out below, ready to add to broth or fruit juice. (The solids remaining in the filter are nonfat yogurt cheese – enjoy it as you would sour cream or cream cheese in spreads and dips.)

Liquid Tips

❧ Keep a cup or pitcher, or thermos jug of water, juice, or broth where your patient can reach it whenever she wants it.

❧ Keep a record. That can help you remember, and also act as a persuader: "Gee, it is already noon, time for your next cup."

❧ For stuffy noses, try drinking apple juice hot, simmered with a clove, a stick of cinnamon, a slice of fresh gingerroot – one or all. The aromatic spices help clear congestion.

❧ Fruit juice tastes good at first, but after awhile something savory seems better. Broth, herb teas, or miso broth are tasty and beneficial.

❧ Clear, diluted apple juice is one of the first things to offer someone who has had any digestive upset. Serve the juice warm, or, at least, not too cold.

❧ If nausea prevents drinking, try small slivers of ice.

❧ Milk is more of a food than a liquid, especially if it becomes concentrated (by long heating, for example). Then, it contains such a lot of protein and minerals that instead of providing fluids, it may have the opposite effect.

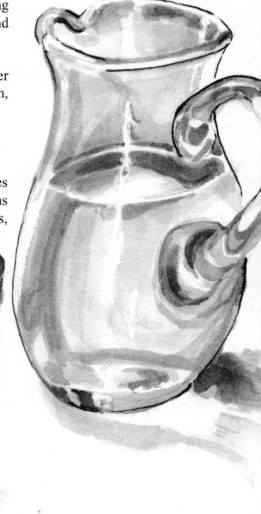
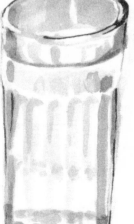

Juices, Some Thoughts

FRUIT JUICE

Fruit juices taste good, and they also provide needed fluid and, sometimes, needed calories. A note of caution, though. Fruit juices contain a lot of (natural) sugar, and sugar can aggravate diarrhea, so when that is the problem, offer broth and herbal teas. If the patient wants fruit juice, best dilute it with water or mineral water.

But what about that sugar? Is it a good idea to offer sweet beverages or food to someone fighting an illness? Folk wisdom says no, and ancient medical systems that we know about also discourage it. If you are one who seems to get the flu every New Year after piling on the Christmas sweets, maybe you're ready to believe there's logic behind a ban. This line of thought has been reinforced in the last year by several reports in the popular press mentioning (but not citing) research to show that consuming ordinary amounts of sugar impairs immune system function in normal people. We tried hard to pin this down, and did turn up a few very small, provocative studies from the 1970s, but nothing you'd call substantial. Almost all of the work relating to sugar focuses on diabetes, which isn't surprising since it is one of the four major causes of death. But one can't help wishing for more scientific interest in *other* interactions of sugar with health; Americans consume an average of over one hundred thirty pounds of sugar per person per year. If it does affect immune function, that could explain a lot of sickness. But we really don't know.

So where does it leave us? Should I give juice to my friend with a cold? From all we have found out we would have to say that, most likely, a few cups over the course of the day won't hurt. But please remember the positive advantages to be gained from hot drinks, from herbal remedies, from vegetable broth. And remember that sick or well, a person who drinks a lot of juice will not be hungry for real food that contains essential nutrients – protein, vitamins, minerals, fiber – absent in even the best fruit juice.

~&~ Acidic juices like orange, grapefruit, or tomato upset iffy stomachs. Dilute them, or save them for later.

~&~ If you are susceptible to urinary infections, regular use of cranberry (or blueberry) juice has been shown to help prevent them. Unsweetened cranberry juice is very sour, and "cocktail" too loaded with sugar for many people to drink every day. Capsules containing dried concentrate are available.

~&~ Raw vegetable juices have a place in therapies for patients who are robust, and have the digestive power to benefit from their intensity. Something more dilute is probably better for someone who is below par. For most illnesses we (again) suggest broth and appropriate herbal teas, at least until the need for soothing and healing is over, and building time begins.

~&~ Vegetable juices have a role when the need for nutrients is keen, and the digestion good. Unfortunately, once again, little scientific research has been reported to guide us in this area. Even so, I will share a true story:

A dear friend developed a big tumor in his throat. Eating anything was difficult so he was losing weight in spite of his best efforts. I read everything I could find, and noticed that someone once got cancer in mice to remit, feeding them carrots. It wasn't very scientific of me, but I got huge bags of organic carrots and started giving Joe a couple of quarts of juice a day. It went down easy, and provided needed calories if nothing else, so he stopped losing weight. I don't know if it helped at all, but the surgeon who took out the tumor said it came out easier than he'd thought it would.

During his recovery, Joe found that vegetable juice like commercial V-8 was the best thing – somehow its saltiness seemed most welcome. He drank a lot of it, and a lot of miso broth (page 81). Ginger Tea (page 78) helped with a nausea problem, and he appreciated Barley Tea too (page 80).

Joe is fine now, and says Hi.

Herbal Perspectives

Herbs and food can't be separated; the experienced cook knows that everything that goes on the plate has properties that affect health. We certainly can't claim to be expert herbalists – there is such a thing! Still, as home cooks we have a few favorite concoctions, which we herewith share with you. First, though, a glimpse of what has gone before, and how it affects where we are and may go from here.

SOME SLICES OF HISTORY

Until the middle of the last century, the wisdom passed from mother to daughter, from trader to mountain man, would have included how to prepare remedies for the ordinary ailments of the particular time and place – where to find the plants, when to pick them, how to preserve and prepare them. A lot of it, you would just know, in the way that we just know how to set an alarm clock or get across a busy street. In those days before concrete, the medicinal plants were commonplace. You'd easily find what you needed for most problems, and if something unusual came up, you'd know who to go to – an aunt or neighbor with more experience who had, perhaps, a little garden of special herbs.

When Europeans came to the Americas, they brought their favorite plants. Many also learned from native healers. A name to conjure with is Samuel Thomson – a thoughtful, brilliant man, he developed safe, effective treatments based on Native American wisdom and techniques. (Simply put, when something goes wrong the thing to do is to encourage the internal healer.) Especially given the primitive state of "regular doctoring" in those days, his ideas gained wide popularity. However, at the turn of the century, Americans were looking not to the past but confidently to the future, and by the early 1900s, "modern" medicine had subsumed all other approaches to healing in the United States.

Shift backward, to England, 1800s. Country people moved to the cities to work in factories. On every street, someone would set up a little shop offering the same herbal remedies the folks who'd moved to that area had used back home in the countryside. These people knew plants. If someone was selling toadflax, it had better be toadflax and not leafy spurge. The customers knew, the retailer knew, the guy who brokered them could tell at a glance.

The herb trade flourished. City life brought new diseases; people tried new remedies. Plants arriving from India, China, and the Americas entered the lists. A book about Thomson's ideas that got published in London quickly went to forty-four printings. By the time the British Medical Association was established, herbalists were strong enough to associate too, and command recognition. They set standards for training and treatment that stood for nearly a century. Almost half of the recommended herbs were American.

This section draws from Simon Y. Mills' The Essential Book of Herbal Medicine *(Penguin, London, 1993), an outstanding introduction to the worlds of herbal medicine.*

Another shift, this time to present-day US. In the space of a decade, millions of people have become interested in buying "alternative" remedies. Our government, unlike England and Europe, has no regulatory standards for herbal remedies, and (in the present anti-regulatory political climate) none in sight. Few of us who use these remedies, cut off as we are from tradition, know what to look for, or what is reasonable to expect from them. We might not know mint from sage, let alone toadflax from leafy spurge, and anyway we buy the herbs in boxes or bottles, trusting that they are what they say they are, trusting that the young woman in the health food store knows what she is talking about when she says goldenseal tea will do the trick.

Admirable companies have sprung up, growing and gathering herbs responsibly, processing them with scrupulous care. Others see a chance to make easy money. These may not see the need to check the bale of roots when it arrives at the dock to determine whether it really is in fact properly dried second-year *dang-gui*. Harvesters, often poor people challenged to find plants to supply the sudden demand that in many areas has depleted normal sources – perhaps gathering in new areas, where plant species differ, and are unfamiliar – sometimes include look-alikes. Middlemen, selling by the ton, think of ways to increase the weight. Who's to know? Insects and rodents leave their contributions. Drying, cutting, sifting, grinding: contaminants enter unnoticed. Compounders, lacking the scarce traditional herb, substitute a little synthetic for the same effect . . . And so it goes: arsenic and amphetamines, belladonna, mercury, lead, valium, and ibuprofen have been found in herbal medications.[1,2] Responsible parties in the burgeoning industry are working to establish standards, but it'll be awhile before there's Law West of the Pecos – or even Cape Cod.

꿍

CAUTIONS

1. Herbs excel in ameliorating everyday problems. They are not appropriate for sole treatment of acute illness.
2. Some herbal preparations, like some medicines, should not be used by pregnant or nursing mothers, infants, or young children.
3. Any medication can be used unwisely. But it's more than that. In this country, the government does not regulate herbs as it does drugs – for dosage, ingredient content, or quality. Inappropriate use and plain carelessness have caused illnesses and deaths.
4. There's a lot of unsubstantiated hype. Some combination preparations have been tested and found to contain little – some, *none* – of claimed herbal ingredients. Be skeptical; use common sense.

Read the label: it should show Latin name of the herbs, address of the actual manufacturer, batch number, date of manufacture, and expiration date. *(Vegetarians: Chinese medicine includes insect and animal parts in the term "herb.")*
Stop taking an herb immediately if you have adverse effects.

1. *"Anticholinergic Poisoning Associated with an Herbal Tea– New York City, 1994," JAMA, April 19, 1995, vol 273, no 15, p. 1166.*

2. *"Relative Safety of Herbal Medicines," Norman R. Farnsworth,* HerbalGram, *Special Supplement no. 29, 1993, p. 36-E – 36-G.*

Where does this leave us? If we are to reclaim this treasurehouse, we need to educate ourselves. There are some books written by people with excellent credentials. Always, it is useful to ask questions of people who have experience – in this case, that seldom means clerks in health food stores, alas. Experiment with simple preparations you're interested in. Try to buy from reputable companies. Grow the herbal plants that you find useful. If you find your interest is increasing, you may want to subscribe to

> *HerbalGram*
> Herb Research Foundation
> 1007 Pearl St., Suite 200
> Boulder, CO 80302

How to know if a company selling herbs is reliable? There are no guarantees. One way to get information about a product is to call the company that makes it. Ask them how long they have been in business. What quality control programs do they have? How do they determine herb identity and potency? How do they protect endangered plant species? Do they belong to a trade organization like the American Herbal Products Association (AHPA), which sets standards for members?

Maybe best of all is familiarity with the fresh herb. "With echinacea," a wise woman told me, "If you just once bite into a fresh root, from then on you can tell about the power of a tincture right away."

The field of herbal medicine grows and changes – this is true even in the hoariest, most extensively articulated traditional systems. Just now, terrific energy fills the world of healing. Bright men and women study not only the methods of their ancestors, but Ayurveda, Chinese medicine, Native American, and African ways of healing. Moreover, they apply what they learn to diseases unknown in other times. There's increasing scientific interest. Probably no one can claim to see the whole picture, but it is not all chaos. Many respected remedies have stood the test of time – and even scientific research. The list that follows is far from complete even as an introduction, but these are remedies we know and use, and they are safe and effective. We also sometimes turn to commercial preparations like echinacea tincture, and find tea bags like "Breathe Easy" and "Throat Coat" helpful and convenient when colds strike. From the Ayurvedic medicine chest, *hingwastika* mercifully alleviates intestinal gas; *triphala* is an effective, yet gentle, laxative.

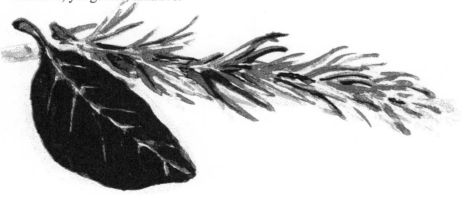

Useful Herbal Remedies & Teas

ALOE VERA

A big window box planted with aloe vera sits right next to our kitchen door. When anyone has a burn or scrape or sting, we cut a succulent aloe leaf, split it open, and apply the inside to the wound. It is wonderfully soothing, and promotes healing. Aloe grows easily in any reasonably sunny place protected from frost. Aloe vera gel in bottles has played to mixed scientific reviews, partly because it is so easy to contaminate. But no one has anything but praise for the fresh leaf.

CHAMOMILE

Unless otherwise noted, the material on these pages is drawn from our own experience, and checked against Varro Tyler's exceedingly useful books, The Honest Herbal *(1993) and* Herbs of Choice *(1994), both from Haworth Press, New York.*

Soothing and calming, chamomile tea is one of the most widely used of all herbal remedies. It gently aids digestion and has anti-inflammatory and anti-infective properties, useful for colds and flu, and externally for scrapes and rashes. Helps reduce menstrual cramps because it reduces spasms. Calming before bed for children and grown-ups alike. Individuals who are very allergic to the Aster family of flowers (ragweed, mums, etc.) should exercise caution, but otherwise, a good choice for everyday drinking. When making tea, pour a cup of boiling water over a heaping tablespoon of flower heads, and steep in a covered vessel for at least 15 minutes to get the most benefit. Easy to grow, inexpensive to buy.

Echinacea is one of the valuable curative plants originally used by the Native Americans. A respected anti-infective agent, it fell into disuse when sulfa drugs came on the scene in the 1930s. Recent research demonstrates that echinacea stimulates the immune system by increasing the activity of white blood cells, and in certain other ways. A few doses of echinacea tincture really do seem to be able to stave off an oncoming cold or flu. Echinacea is also useful externally to promote wound healing. No toxicity has been reported, but if you want it to work for you when you need it, don't take it all the time.

This beautiful perennial "grows like a weed" for some people but, so far, not in our gardens! However, the tincture is available wherever herbal preparations are sold, and tincture is the preferred vehicle because some active constituents are more readily absorbed.

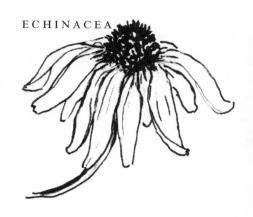

ECHINACEA

Ephedra is a sparse, stemmy desert plant used in cold remedies for thousands of years because it so effectively relieves nasal congestion and bronchial constriction.

Recently, irresponsible companies have misused ephedra by including it, concentrated to toxic levels, in preparations sold for weight loss, or for an herbal "high," and there have been tragic consequences. Ephedra contains the powerful alkaloids ephedrine and pseudoephedrine, which have pharmacological action similar to adrenaline (epinephrine). *Use a reasonable amount (see margin). Do not give to anyone for whom the drug ephedrine would be counterindicated: those with high blood pressure, heart disease, thyroid disease, diabetes, prostate enlargement; to anyone who is pregnant or nursing, or taking anti-depressants.*

American varieties of ephedra (for example, Mormon Tea) do not contain the powerful alkaloid compound, and are used mainly as a slightly bitter beverage.

EPHEDRA
(MA HUANG)

Reality check:
A tea prepared by pouring
1 cup boiling water over
1 heaping teaspoonful
ma huang herb
and steeping 10 minutes,
yields a drink with
15-30 mg of ephedrine.
(Herbs of Choice p. 89)

Over-the-counter allergy tablets usually have 30 (or 60) mg ephedrine.

LICORICE Many cough remedies include licorice root because it is soothing, an effective expectorant, and tastes sweet and lovely. Cough lozenges and candies with licorice in them do help a sore throat. In the US, you need to check the label to see whether the product really is licorice – in this country, most "licorice" is flavored with anise oil. One reason for this is that licorice raises blood pressure, especially in sensitive people. Heroic amounts of real licorice candy, and lesser amounts of licorice consumed over a period of time, have precipitated serious illnesses, and even deaths. As with many things, a little can indeed be helpful, but more isn't better.

Some particularly delicious herbal tea blends, incidentally, contain licorice root; enjoy them, but not every day.

LINDEN Calming linden flower tea tastes pleasant, and is good any time. Linden gently promotes sweating, and so is helpful in fever.

VALERIAN A respected, safe and effective tranquillizer and sedative, used to promote sleep for over a thousand years. Prepare tea with a rounded teaspoonful of herb per cup, and take at bedtime. Safe to use several times a day, if needed. It does smell pretty bad, so a lot of people find the tincture easier to use (half a teaspoonful). No side effects or toxic reactions have ever been reported

It is important that the herb be fresh, or if used in tincture, that it have been prepared with care. We can't entirely recommend growing your own: valerian is reputed to be attractive to rats, and some say that is what the Pied Piper used to get them to follow him out of Hameln.

WHITE WILLOW BARK *contains an aspirin-like ingredient and can be effective, but should* NOT *be given to children who have any kind of viral fever like flu or chickenpox – just as aspirin shouldn't.*

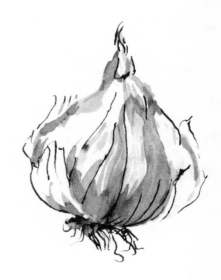

Kitchen Herbs & Spices

As we have noted elsewhere, the ordinary herbs and spices used in cooking have medicinal properties. Of course, *all* foods have properties that influence our well-being in one direction or the other – hence the wise saying, "Food is your best medicine."

Aromatics like cinnamon, ginger, and cloves, and also thyme and sage, included in hot drinks, help relieve congestion – as we mention elsewhere.

Not surprisingly, a chief effect of culinary spices is to aid digestion. Among these, particular helpers are cumin (Mexican chili beans, Indian curries), fennel (Italian sauces, soups), mustard (ubiquitous in Indian cooking, and not unknown here at home); ginger (see next page), chili, coriander seed. The coriander plant's green leaves are also beneficial, and appear in Indian vegetable and grain preparations, in Latin American dishes – a.k.a. *cilantro* – and in Chinese cooking too ("Chinese parsley"). Gentle, sweetly aromatic cardamom, most familiar in the West as the warm, bright flavor in Scandinavian bakery specialties, comes from India, where it's used in sweets and as an ingredient in *garam masala*. Even good old black pepper "ignites the digestive fire."

These spices do help promote a healthy digestion. In illness, however, and for certain individuals, mildly flavored foods are more soothing.

ॐ

Fennel seed deserves special mention as an anti-flatulent. Steep a teaspoon in simmering water to make tea; or, in the Indian way, toast the seeds lightly and chew a pinch after the meal. Other members of the fennel family offer similar benefit: for example, caraway, often added to cabbage dishes and heavy rye breads in Eastern European cooking; and cumin, such a helpful addition to beans.

FENNEL

Garlic has been used medicinally for many centuries. Today, most authorities testify to its effectiveness at fighting germs, lowering blood pressure and cholesterol, reducing the tendency of the blood to clot, and helping prevent some cancers. It has been extensively studied; more than a thousand papers have been published on garlic in the last twenty years alone. Even so, in June of 1996, *The University of California at Berkeley Wellness Letter* reported on their own researchers' careful examination of the gigantic body of research on garlic. They found that the studies of garlic's effects have been flawed, and have produced contradic-

GARLIC

tory results. Their conclusion: "No clear evidence that garlic has any health benefits." Well, the jury *may* be out, but . . .

For believers, some further information: Allicin, one primary active component, is produced in *raw* garlic when it is crushed. Allicin and other beneficial compounds are destroyed in cooking. Ordinary garlic powder has about the same activity as supplements in pills, but since stomach acid inactivates some beneficial properties, enteric-coated capsules that dissolve not in the stomach but in the intestines are more likely to deliver their payload. These have the added advantage of minimizing odor.

GINGER

Ginger Tea is a standby for us. We like it any time, with honey or plain. Very helpful to relieve a mild stomachache or headache, or for nausea, colds, or fever. Turn the page for some Ginger Tea recipes we like very much.

Ginger is called the "universal medicine" in India.[3] In China, it is "the doctor" – so esteemed that it is used in fully half of all medicinal herbal combinations.[4] Scientific studies continue to come along verifying many of the virtues tradition credits ginger with possessing, among them its efficacy against nausea and vomiting, and its usefulness as a digestive aid. (Indian friends say that you would never serve a rich feast without including a gingery chutney to help digest it.) In addition, ginger helps promote sweating and reduces fever, relieves coughs, and gently soothes pain. There have been no reports of toxicity.

In counteracting nausea, ginger acts on the digestive system, not the central nervous system or the inner ear, making it safe to use even in pregnancy.[5] However, ginger *is* an anti-coagulant, so if you are taking medication that affects the ability of your blood to clot, do not make big changes in how much ginger you use without consulting your doctor.

Ginger ale and crystallized ginger can be convenient forms of ginger to keep on hand for car trips. Both have enough of ginger's active principles to be effective.

GINGER AND HONEY: Grate fresh gingerroot and squeeze it to extract juice – with your fingers or in a garlic press. Most of the juice comes off the back of the press. Lift the pulp and squeeze a couple of times. Mix the juice with honey to taste, and give it neat, right off the spoon, for sore throat or cough.

3. David Frawley and Vasant Lad, The Yoga of Herbs. (Lotus Press, Santa Fe, NM, 1986), p. 122.

4. Steven Foster and Yue Chongxi, Herbal Emissaries. (Healing Arts Press, Rochester, VT, 1992), p. 95ff.

5. "Ginger as an Anti-nausea Remedy in Pregnancy: The Issue of Safety," HerbalGram 38, Winter 1996, pp. 47–50.

Mint grows enthusiastically in any partially sunny place that gets some water. The pretty green leaves smell wonderful if you brush the plant as you walk by. When I was a little girl I used to like to go and sit quietly by myself near my grandma's mint patch – the very air was tonic.

To make tea, pour boiling water over a sprig in a cup, or use dried leaves, or a mint tea bag. My grandma used to add brown sugar and plenty of milk for us kids, but the tea is good plain too, or with honey. Besides spearmint, gardeners can give you flavors like orange, pineapple, bergamot, even chocolate! All taste good, and make a bracing hot drink that is welcome anytime, especially when you have a cold. Our top favorite variety of mint is Anise Hyssop. Combined with honey, it's a mild, effective expectorant. But the flavor is too lovely to relegate only to cold season! The leaves make the best, best herb tea, and the tiny purple flowers, sprinkled in salad, give a wonderful sweet, peppery spark.

Incidentally, *peppermint* is the one that relieves digestive complaints. Other mints do not have the menthol content that makes peppermint so settling to the stomach. The same ingredient makes peppermint tea too strong for very young children.

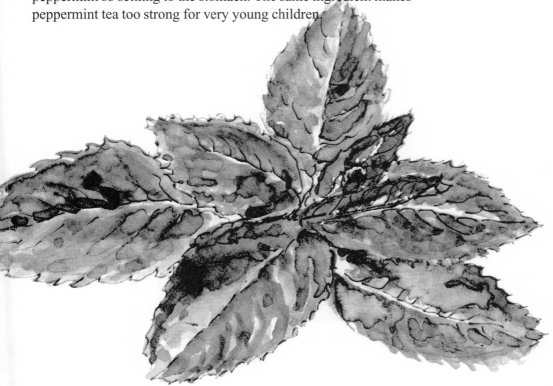

Ginger Tea

1 quart water
2" nub of gingerroot

Set water to boil in a saucepan. Peel and thinly slice the ginger-root. Drop it into the boiling water and simmer for 10 minutes or more, until the flavor seems just right to you. Strain and serve plain, or with honey, or honey and milk. Ginger Tea can become too strong, in which case it irritates instead of soothing. If it seems strong to you, thin it down with water. Cool, and keep in a jar in the refrigerator for a few days, to serve cold, or reheat as needed.

JAL JEERA: While heating the water as for Ginger Tea, dry-roast ¼ teaspoon of cumin seeds until they darken just a shade and give you their fragrance. Add to the water along with the ginger, and proceed as above for Ginger Tea. Adjust the proportions to suit your taste.

TEA OF THE GOOD YOUNG PRINCE: Soothing and clearing. Brew Ginger Tea. When you turn off the heat, add a tablespoon of fennel seed and ¼ teaspoon of coarsely ground cardamom seeds. Cover and let cool to drinking temperature. Strain. Very good indeed, plain or with honey, warm or cold.

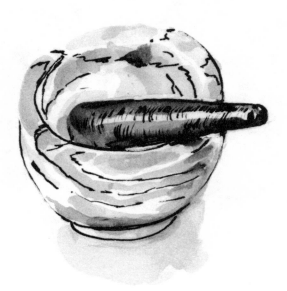

Karen's Tea

We make this magical tea to help clear a stuffy head and soothe a sore throat. It is very good tasting all by itself, but if you like, add fresh lemon juice and honey – both do help soothe sore throats.

10 cups water in a pan with a lid

1 tablespoon echinacea root
1 tablespoon dandelion root
1 tablespoon blackberry root

1–2 tablespoons marshmallow root
1 tablespoon ephedra leaf

1 tablespoon mullein leaf
2–3 tablespoons peppermint leaf
1–2 tablespoons elder flower
1 tablespoon catnip

Boil water; reduce heat, and stir in the first 3 tough roots. Cover loosely, and simmer gently 10 minutes. Add the next 2 sturdy herbs, and simmer as before, another 10 minutes.

Now, remove the pan from the heat and add the tender leaves. Cover and allow to steep away from the heat 10 more minutes.

Strain and serve. Store the extra in jars in the refrigerator to heat gently as needed.

Because of the ephedra, limit the amount taken in one day to one batch; less for a child – or omit the ephedra.

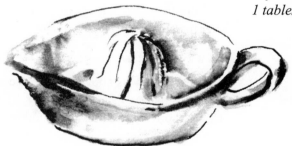

Lemon & Honey

A family recipe from so many Moms! Delicious and effective. Squeeze a lemon and stir in honey in an approximately equal amount, to taste; then add boiling water to make a cup. Sip to soothe a sore throat.

Can also serve the lemon and honey undiluted, off the spoon.

Barley Tea

2 quarts boiling water
½ cup organic barley,
    whole-grain "naked" or
    hulled, but not pearl
3 cardamom pods
    (or ¼ teaspoon ground
    cardamom)

Soothing, warming, bright-tasting, healing, and building. Simply wonderful for anyone with weakness, irritated digestive tract, sore throat. Worth the price of the book for this alone.

Boil water in a large saucepan. Wash the barley in cold water and drain it. Put it into the boiling water, and simmer actively about half an hour, until the water is a lovely deep pink, and cloudy. Either strain it, or let it stand, and then pour off the clear liquid. If desired, you can add another quart of water to the barley, and boil again, combining the liquid from both. You should end up with about 8 cups of barley tea – but you can make it stronger or more dilute, as you wish.

With mortar and pestle, grind seeds from cardamom pods quite fine, and add to the hot tea. Serve hot with honey or sugar if wanted.

Store the extra in the refrigerator to heat whenever you need it over the next couple of days.

BARLEY CHAI

a big cinnamon stick
½ teaspoon whole black
    peppercorns
2 cloves
1 teaspoon fennel seed, or
    star anise
about 6 slices fresh
    gingerroot

Proceed exactly as above, adding the spices to the pan when you put in the barley.
This is more stimulating than soothing.

TWO OBSERVATIONS

The beautiful pink color sometimes plays hard-to-get. Pinkness doesn't affect the taste of the tea or its beneficial qualities, but the color is so lovely that it's worth going to a little extra trouble to get. Make sure the water is at a rolling boil when you put in the grain. Rinse the grain *just* before, in *cold* water.

The used-up barley grains have given their goodness to the broth. If you find it hard to throw them away, tasting some will convince you that the compost heap may indeed be the best place for them – like coffee grounds.

Miso Broth

Hot miso broth has a deep salty-savory taste that's extra welcome when you have a cold. If you are not already familiar with miso's hearty flavor, prepare to find yourself liking it so much that you include it in your routine after you are well too, as a daily, nearly instant hot drink.

Miso occupies a place of honor in classical Japanese cuisine. Its proponents believe that miso goes beyond flavor to actually promoting health, and an impressive amount of modern research has substantiated these claims. Produced by fermenting soybeans and grains, the miso you buy may be pasteurized, but if it isn't, it contains active cultures antagonistic to microbes that cause common diseases. Like yogurt, unpasteurized miso requires proper storage and should be used within the specified time.

❧

Make broth by mixing a few teaspoons of miso, to taste, into a cup of hot water. To get the benefit of the active cultures, buy fresh miso rather than "instant," and stir it into your cup just before you drink it. There are many kinds and flavors to try, and beyond the simple broth we have described, literally hundreds of soups for which miso makes the base. If you are interested in knowing more about this fascinating, useful, and delicious food, please read *The Book of Miso* by William Shurtleff and Akiko Aoyagi.

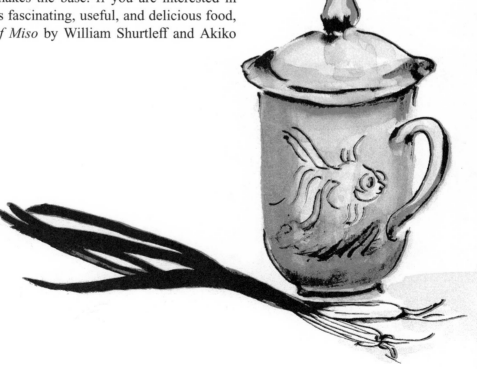

Gentle Vegetable Broth

Tried-and-true; a versatile, delicious, and simple concoction.

*2 small zucchini
  or use winter squash,
    potatoes, or carrot
handful green beans
handful parsley stems
  or spinach stems
big pinch salt
2 quarts cold water*

*1 cup parsley
  and/or spinach leaves*

FOR SAD TUMS: Ideal sipping to soothe digestive upset, or any time the innards are not yet perfectly settled.

Wash and cut up the vegetables. Put all the ingredients except the leaves in a saucepan and simmer gently about 20 minutes, until the vegetables are soft. Add the leaves and simmer 10 minutes more, then drain. Discard the vegetables. Serve soon, cooling and refrigerating what is left, but use within a day or two.

FOR COLDS: When the *digestion* is just fine, but *congestion* is a problem, add to the above, from the start: onion, garlic, toasted cumin seed, red or black pepper, pinch of thyme.

The steaming cup with its aromatic ingredients helps you clear from the first whiff to the last swallow.

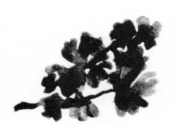

FOR FEVER: Add warming herbs: ginger, or basil, sage, and thyme.

One Delicious Broth

This is a no-excuses, deluxe broth. Even so, if you lack some ingredient, any logical substitute will do fine. The thing to aim for is a balance of tart/savory and sweet vegetables; a couple of corn cobs (corn cut off), a handful of pea pods (no peas), or a slice of winter squash – these count in on the sweet side. Asparagus, spinach, more parsley, bay leaves, etc., weigh on the other side.

Leave out cabbagey vegetables (kale, broccoli, cauliflower, turnips, etc.); they give a sulfury taste, and can cause gas.

๑

Chop the onion and cut up the vegetables.

Heat the oil in an 8-quart pot and add the onion and garlic, the whole spices and yellow split peas, and stir and sauté until a lovely golden brown. Add the rest of the ingredients except the parsley. Bring to a boil, then turn down the heat and simmer gently until the vegetables are soft. Add the parsley, cover, and remove from heat. Let cool. Pour off the broth, straining out and discarding everything else. Correct for salt.

Makes 3 or 4 heavenly quarts.

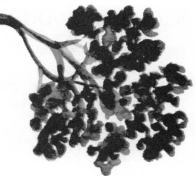

a large onion
several cloves garlic
oil to sauté
handful yellow split peas
tablespoon cumin seeds
*2 tablespoons coriander
 seeds*

*2" nub of gingerroot,
 peeled and chopped*
½ teaspoon turmeric
2 potatoes
*4 inside stalks of celery,
 including leaves*
3 carrots
3 zucchini
big handful green beans
*2 red ripe tomatoes, seeds
 removed*
big handful barley, not pearl
2 teaspoons salt
teaspoon black peppercorns
*2 stalks curry leaves, or a
 small bay leaf*
6 quarts water

big handfuls parsley

Golden Broth

1 onion, chopped
1 clove garlic
½ cup yellow split peas
2 tablespoons oil

½ teaspoon turmeric
2 quarts hot water
½ teaspoon salt

Laurel's Kitchen correspondents swear by Golden Broth as a vegetarian stand-in wherever chicken stock is called for.

Sauté onion, whole garlic, and peas in oil until delicately brown. Stir in turmeric and add water and salt. Simmer together at least half an hour. Strain for a thin stock, purée for a thick one.

VARIATIONS

Sautéing at the start, as above, allows you to strain the solids out to make a clear stock, but if you want to omit that step, just boil all the ingredients together – the results will be thick and good, with or without the oil.
Green Broth: Substitute green splits for the yellow. Add a bay leaf and omit the turmeric.

Golden Noodle Soup

2 quarts clear Golden Broth
big handful whole wheat
    ribbon noodles
1 cup each diced celery,
    potatoes, carrots
1 teaspoon salt
½ cup finely chopped
    parsley

Our triumphant answer to Ma Campbell and to all the colds, malaises, and depressions that are usually soothed from corporate cans. This wonderful, elemental, satisfying soup does it all at least as well, and it is easy, too. And cheap.

If you have Golden Broth already, bring it to a boil and add everything else except the parsley. Simmer gently about half an hour, until the vegetables are tender. Add the parsley and adjust the salt.

If you haven't already made the broth, here is a shortcut. Make the broth in one pot, reducing the liquid by about half. Bring a quart of water to boil in a second pot, and simmer the noodles and vegetables in that. Combine them after you purée or strain the broth. (Cooking the peas together with the vegetables lengthens the cooking time for the peas, for some reason.) Total cooking time is just over half an hour.

Sometimes we add chopped chard, or spinach, tomatoes, or broccoli near the end of cooking time.

Makes about 10 cups of soup. You won't be sorry.

Fragrant Tomato Broth

In India, it is said that the herb coriander is so beneficial, there is no ailment which it does not ameliorate. Here is a delicious red brothy soup whose flavor is lifted invisibly by the bracing herb.

Fresh ripe tomatoes make a difference here. For better flavor with less-than-perfect tomatoes, use broth instead of water, or choose one of the ginger versions below.

1 onion, chopped
2 whole cloves garlic
2 tablespoons olive oil

6 red ripe tomatoes, chopped
* (or 2–3 cups canned)*
2 cups broth or water
salt and black pepper to
* taste*

1 bunch fresh coriander
* (cilantro)*

๛

Sauté onion and garlic in oil. Add the tomatoes, and broth or water. Bring to a boil, stirring occasionally, and simmer for about 10 minutes. Wash and add the unchopped coriander, and simmer another 10 minutes. Strain, discarding the pulp and herb.

Taste for salt. If you used salty broth or canned tomatoes, additional salt may be unnecessary.

VARIATIONS

↪ Use a packed ½ cup of fresh basil leaves, or 2 tablespoons dried basil, instead of coriander.

↪ For colds, add a bit of red chili with the onion.

↪ *For a thicker soup:* As above; except don't chop the tomatoes; halve them, and shake out the seeds. Holding the skin side, grate on a cheese/vegetable grater, allowing the pulp to fall in a bowl. Add this pulp to the pan when the onion and garlic are golden. Discard the tomato skins and seeds. Cook as described, removing the coriander with tongs before serving.

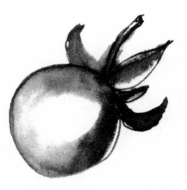

Gingery Tomato Soup

Proceed as above, stirring in a tablespoon of minced gingerroot when you have nearly finished sautéing the onion and garlic. Add shoyu/tamari to taste. Omit coriander, or add some chopped leaves when you serve. Excellent for colds.

FAST AND EASY: Use canned puréed tomatoes, and skip the blending step. (This version can double as a tasty light sauce for rice or baked potatoes.)

We use a lot of tomatoes year-round – maybe you do, too. Whether canned or fresh, commercial tomatoes have an especially high level of pesticide residues. This is a good place to go for organic when you can.

Was It a Virus – or What?

Was that "flu" actually food poisoning? Symptoms are often similar. Both can come from unwashed hands. Food poisoning is easy to prevent with good habits.

If you are caring for someone who is frail, debilitated, or has a compromised immune system, you know that these suggestions are even more important.

✌ Bacteria that cause food poisoning live on hands, in the air, on countertops and chopping boards. Washing helps a lot. You can't eliminate them completely, but reducing their numbers makes a big difference. Healthy people can fight off a few microbes; sick people find it harder. No one can beat millions.

✌ Think like a microbe! Germs that live and cause trouble in our bodies thrive in body-like environments. Keep alert for the cozy conditions that microbe families thrive in: food that's soft and moist. Not too hot, not too cold, not sour, or fiercely sweet or salty. Sandwich fixings, oh, boy! Potato or macaroni salad, yeah. Lukewarm casseroles, leftovers – way to GO! And, ah, yes, creamy fillings in pastries . . . classic breeding grounds for food poisoning! How so? They've been handled (bacteria installed), so when these *middley* foods are left at *middley* temperatures, germs multiply like crazy.

SOME TIPS

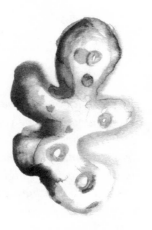

Wash your hands and kitchen surfaces with attention and thoroughly. If you have flesh foods in your kitchen, keep separate chopping boards, and bleach them often.

In the refrigerator: When you put leftovers away, use shallow containers. Be sure there's plenty of room for air circulation around them so that they can cool quickly, and not warm up the items near them. Use a thermometer to check your refrigerator. It should be between 33° and 40°F, and not stuffed to the gills.

Just assume eggs and flesh foods are contaminated. Wipe up that streak of egg white between the bowl and the sink strainer before someone puts a bagel down in it. No one, especially children, should taste raw batter that has egg in it.

Remember the middley rule of thumb: "2:40/140". Don't serve or eat food that has been left more than 2 hours at temperatures above 40° or below 140°F.

First Foods After Digestive Upset

After nausea and vomiting quiet down, the first thing to offer is sips of water. If your sickie can't deal even with water, offer slivers of ice to suck.

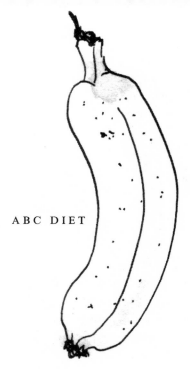

ABC DIET

ҙᴑ When he feels ready to drink something, first give diluted clear liquids like apple juice, weak tea, mild clear broth, whichever sounds good to him.

ҙᴑ When fluids stay down, go to "A B C": applesauce, banana, cream of rice. Rice is preferred to wheat, because its starch is more digestible. Fat-free rice crackers are good. Brown rice is rougher than white, wait on that.

ҙᴑ If these sit well, offer plain, peeled baked or boiled potatoes, tapioca, then other gentle foods: saltine crackers, dry toast. Applesauce would be better for topping than butter.

ҙᴑ

Fat can challenge a recovering digestive system. Wait to see how the patient feels; meantime go easy on the butter for that potato.

SOME TIPS

Milk should be reintroduced slowly after severe diarrhea, which can temporarily suspend the gut's production of the enzyme lactase (which helps digest milk). Drinking milk again too soon may seem to cause a relapse.

A nondairy shake: blend a ripe, but not over- ripe, banana with a cup of soymilk – nourishing and digestible for most everyone.

Gas-causing foods: Everyone's different. Your patient will probably be able to say right off what is likely to cause trouble. Some of the usual suspects: carbonated beverages, beans, cabbage-family vegetables; bread; pasta; raw apples, pears, peaches; prunes, corn, oats, potatoes, bran; strong-flavored or spicy food; alcohol, caffeine.

After the digestion settles, serve yogurt or other products containing beneficial live cultures. A healthy person's gut is home to many species of beneficial microbes. There is substantial evidence that traditional cultured products like yogurt and miso, and certain other fermented foods, encourage these helpful little guys.

BACK TO NORMAL

Applesauce & Stewed Apples

6 apples
apple juice, or water
(sweetener)

A welcome delicacy, in all its manifestations. A perfect first food after digestive upset, first served plain, then over cream of rice or cottage cheese. Freshly made applesauce is just great, any time or place.

ॐ

FOR STEWED APPLES: Peel and core the apples and cut them into attractive chunks. Place in a saucepan and pour juice over them until it is about an inch deep in the pan. Bring to a boil and simmer uncovered until the fruit is soft, stirring once or twice to insure against sticking. Check sweetness and add sugar or the sweetener you prefer, if it is needed.

FOR APPLESAUCE: As above, but mash the cooked fruit with a fork, or spin it in the blender. A quick route to applesauce is to cook the quartered fruit without peeling, then put it through a food mill.

ॐ

VARIATIONS, FANCIES

Raisins cooked with the fruit provide interesting texture and enough added sweetness for most apples.
Adding a stick of cinnamon gives bright flavor without the disagreeable catching in the throat that the ground spice may cause.
For a sophisticated nip, add a long thin slice of fresh gingerroot with, or instead of, the cinnamon, taking it out when the flavor seems strong enough to you. Both cinnamon and ginger, as we have said elsewhere, help ameliorate sore throats and congestion.

My Grandma's Applesauce

Core and peel organically grown apples, putting the peels and cores, but not the ends, in a saucepan. Cover them with water and cook until soft. Strain, discarding the peels and saving the broth. Meantime, while the peels simmer, cut the apples into quarters, then the quarters in half. Put them into the strained apple broth, and cook until apples are soft. My grandma used quite a bit of sugar, she being Pennsylvania Dutch, but that's another story. With or without sugar, you'll be impressed how much better it tastes this way, and once you get used to doing it, it doesn't take any longer, either.

Astonishing Applesauce

If you can find or grow them, use ripe, rosy "Pink Pearl" apples, so pretty and so delicious. Peel and cook the apples, and blend them smooth in the blender. This delicate, custardy applesauce, bright deep pink, defies description, but you won't be disappointed!

Stewed Pears

Make stewed pears like apples, using gingerroot, a cinnamon stick, or lemon peel for added flavor. For a pretty effect, cook a handful of dried cranberries along with the pears.

Tapioca

Tapioca is gentle, very good for building up again after digestive problems. Convalescents for whom milk is acceptable will welcome regular old-fashioned tapioca pudding made according to the directions on the box. Please note, though, at least today as we go to print, the text on the box still offers a variation that calls for uncooked egg whites. Because it is no longer safe to use egg that has not been thoroughly cooked – even unbroken eggs have been found to contain salmonella bacteria – stick to the recipe that calls for cooking the eggs.

TAILORING THE RECIPE

- *Without egg:* If you follow the box's recipe simply omitting the egg, you will get a thin dotty liquid. Thicken it nicely by spinning ½ cup of the liquid and its dots in the blender. Return the thick, smooth result to the pot of pudding. Without the egg, the pudding is less rich in fat and much blander in flavor.

- *Without dairy:* Substitute soymilk for milk (and egg). Or, use apple juice for the liquid measure, omitting egg and sweetener. This gives a bland applesauce-like pudding, a very useful first food for a child, especially after a bout of diarrhea. Add a cinnamon stick and a handful of raisins to the pot to make a more interesting dish for a healthy digester.

See pages 47 and 132 also – and try Gummy-fruit Pudding just for fun . . .

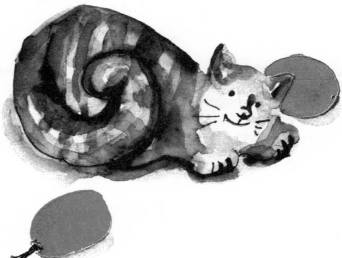

Gummy-fruit Pudding

This wonderful stuff is unlike anything you may have run into. In spite of the strange consistency (or because of that?) people do love it.

½ cup medium pearl tapioca*
2 cups fruit juice

ᵹ

Choose clear sweet juice with intense flavor – for sure, not the kind called "nectar." You can also intensify the flavor with such things as cinnamon or ginger, as suggested below.

*Pearl tapioca is available in many natural foods stores.

Soak tapioca in fruit juice for about 4 hours (or more, or overnight in the refrigerator – at least until the pearls have taken up about 1½ cup of the liquid). Put it all in the top of a double boiler and cover, simmering very gently for 3 hours, or until the white dots disappear. Do not boil. Boiling will make it stringy, which goes beyond strange into the twilight zone of weirdness.

For digestions that are more robust, you can intensify the flavor by adding a stick of cinnamon for apple juice, or slices of fresh or candied ginger with pear. Raspberry juice needs no help, and cranberry. . . . Depending on the fruit juice, and your eaters, you may want to adjust the flavor with lemon juice or added sweetener.

Suggested alternate names, depending on your audience: Asteroid Pudding, Polka-dot Pudding.

ᵹ

As above, except cook uncovered, permitting considerable evaporation.

ASTEROID GOO

Pour the resulting thick goo into a glass 9″ × 13″ pan and chill. Cut into gummy squares when cold – fun to eat. I want to say kids love this (which they do, unless they are about four), but grownups are the ones who seem to take a giddy delight in it.

Made with apple juice, this is an excellent first food after diarrhea, it soothes and builds, no toxins or allergies.

Caution: eating really a lot can be constipating, and its subtle deliciousness could possibly tempt you to that.

Home Remedies . . .

These useful standbys may not fit exactly in any section, but they are so effective it would be a shame to leave them out on that account. Let's start with ice.

Ice

For sore muscles, sprains, strains, and spasms, or to areas painful from arthritis, cold packs often provide impressive relief. You can also alternate applications of cold and heat from a heating pad or hot-water bottle. Don't use heat if there's any swelling though.

⮞ For a gentle source of cold, hold a bag of frozen peas on the painful area for 20 minutes. The bag of peas conforms to the shape of the sore place, and peas aren't quite so cold as normal ice. You can turn the bag over at the halfway point. Stop after 20 minutes, but you can repeat several times a day if it helps. Keep the used pea bag in the freezer to use another time, labeled so you will remember not to use these oft-defrosted peas for food.

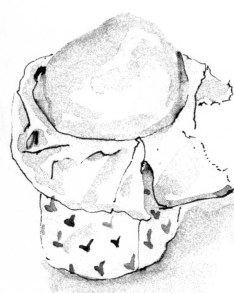

⮞ For deeper pain relief, ice massage can be very helpful. Use an ice cube, or, for your own convenience, freeze water in 4-ounce paper cups (inexpensive "bathroom cups"). Turn down the paper to expose about half an inch of ice; the paper gives you a good grip and prevents you from freezing your fingers. Gently stroke the sore area with the exposed ice for 8 or 10 minutes. For sensitive spots, use the bag of frozen peas for a few minutes beforehand to reduce the shock of the ice, which is much colder. Be sure to tuck towels around the area you are massaging to catch those too-cold trickles!

⮞ Some injuries may respond well to a 20-minute (maximum) application of crushed ice in a bag. Be sure to wrap the ice bag in a damp towel to protect the skin from frostbite. You can even wring the towel out with *warm* water to start the treatment most gently.

Nevermore Nausea Powder

A gift from the ancient Ayurvedic tradition. Tastes good even when you feel queasy. Effective for many people, and safe.

≈

Combine. Chew a little bit, slowly, as often as wanted.

4 teaspoons ginger powder
1 tablespoon coriander powder
½ teaspoon ground cardamom
2 tablespoons brown sugar

Prune Rumble

For drowsy bowels, try this tasty brew. Thin enough to go through a straw. Serve gently warm, or cool.

≈

Blend all ingredients smooth in electric blender; a small blender jar makes this easier. Add hot water to fill a cup, and serve warm. (It will go through a drinking straw if blended smooth enough.)

   Delicious variations: substitute carrot or orange juice for most of the water. Or buttermilk.

3 to 5 stewed prunes (pits gone) and their juice, to cover
juice of one lemon
hot water to make a cup

Gargle

A simple gargle of warm salt water relieves the discomfort of a sore throat, reduces swelling, and removes mucus that causes throat irritation. Just stir ¼ teaspoon of salt into an 8-ounce glass of warm water, stir, and gargle.

¼ teaspoon salt
1 cup warm water

Making It Work

If you are looking after someone with an acute or chronic illness, both of you will benefit so much by learning what you can about it – consult appropriate health professionals, check to see what is in the library or on the Internet. Once you start looking, you'll probably be amazed to see how much relevant information you find – in fact, the challenge then may be making wise choices among a number of possible treatments. Please discuss all the alternatives with your physician, even – no, *particularly* – if you aren't sure she will approve of some of them.

Once you decide to try a course of action, give it full enthusiasm. Your attitude as caregiver, as well as the attitude of the patient greatly influence how effectively the medication or treatment will do its work. Set out confidently, expecting the best. Celebrate every sign of improvement even while you stay alert for problems – especially when you have reason to know that a needed medication may have adverse side effects. Be sure that the medication is taken right on time, carefully following instructions so that it will have its best chance to succeed.

Support a positive frame of mind in every way you can. Give chosen remedies importance and respect in graceful ways – perhaps keep them in a special place on a tray, or in a carved box. Maybe reserve a beautiful glass to use for taking pills. If appropriate, say a short grace together beforehand, then write the time in your record book.

The body has unimaginable healing powers. In some cases, the period of treatment may be partly a way to make a space to rest while the healing happens.

Not everything pans out. An alert caregiver will be ready with another plan.

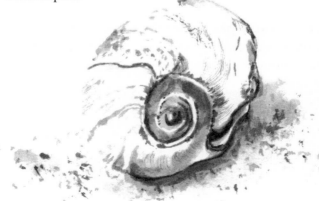

Hospital & Home

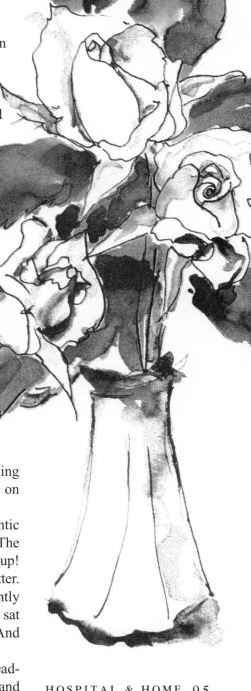

Even when someone seems hopelessly ill, they can get better. In the past few years, three of our friends have had dear family members who seemed impossibly sick, but have recovered wonderfully. One of them was my mom.

When we two daughters arrived at the hospital, she had already been there for days – Daddy hadn't phoned us because he didn't want to call until he had *good* news. Mom was going bananas being so constrained (more literally, restrained). Flat on her back for so long, with half a dozen tubes coming in and going out, her restlessness and anguish were obvious, continuous, unrelieved, and most distressing. Mentally weirded out – so many heavy medications, and ICU is such a noisy moonscape of an environment, no natural rhythms, no day or night. Her sleep was interrupted every half-minute (I counted) by some mechanical noise or procedure. The blood pressure cuff pinched and hissed every five minutes; the IV tube ticked out its automated medication countdown, EKG sensors poking here and there, heart catheter, oxygen cannula and mask, urinary catheter. Peeps and beeps and gurgles and hisses from the machines, groans and sometimes shrieks from adjacent cubicles, nurses chatting with each other about their weekends, family members of other patients rushing by, sobbing or quarreling. Who could blame her for yanking on the tubes, wanting to go home!

Still, incredibly, slowly, day by day, she improved. The frantic restlessness subsided, the blood pressure began to stabilize. The confusion got less. One day when we arrived, she was sitting up! It took two weeks instead of a few days, but she did get better. Daddy, who had been there all those days and nights, gallantly claims the turnaround began when we arrived. I can't say. We sat with her, quietly saying the mantram for long, lovely times. And now she is well, really well. It truly is a miracle.

The mantram is such a help, a caregiver's best friend – it steadies you, it steadies them, it tunes you to a healing wavelength, and it never lets you down. I can't know how much it helped my Mom. It did seem to. But I do know that those hours I spent sitting there holding her hand and silently, heartfully, repeating it, were some of the loveliest, and some of the shortest, hours in my life.

We need always to remember that even when the situation seems hopeless, a person can heal, so hold onto faith, and be ready to help take the next step to help, whatever it is. Healing can be profound even if the person does not get well. Sometimes the next step is to let go.

჻

Another Story

When someone is in the hospital, we tend to think they are in a sort of cocoon with all their needs taken care of. We think, probably it doesn't much matter whether we visit or not. A friend who is a nurse *and* a doctor, says it matters a lot. She says that when someone comes to visit in the hospital bringing quiet optimism, calm and good humor, appreciation for the staff, a willingness to do little comforting things to help – or to just *be* there – it helps the patient, and it also helps the nurses and doctors, "in several ways."

Sometimes it goes beyond this. Sometimes a family member can see something important that the doctors and nurses haven't noticed.

Penelope's mother had been ill for a couple of years, and in and out of the hospital. But this time, Penelope wasn't prepared for what she saw. Her mother was not able to eat the hospital fare at all, and she was getting weaker and weaker. Penelope began bringing things from home, juices, mashed fruits, pudding, soups. Mom began getting a little better. Although medically she was not treatable, she wanted to go home, and she wanted to live. Penelope persuaded the doctors to insert a feeding tube, and they went home together. After that, Mom took her "meals" through the tube. It may have been formula from a can, but it was gourmet "comfort food" nevertheless, served with such love, and it nourished Mom for a precious several months – precious for the family, and crucial for her. She wanted so much to live.

At home, Penelope's mom rejoiced in the beautiful changes of summertime and autumn in the countryside she loved so much.

She participated to the extent she could in the family life around her – all the while taking her time to come to the realization that she could not continue in that body. When she was ready, there was no more holding on. Two days later she left, with purpose, courage, and grace.

Penelope treasures the memory of those months. She watched in wonder as her mother prepared herself step-by-step to face her death. There was a lot of pain. There were problems to solve. At first, eight-year-old Suji and Grandma vied for attention, and that was pretty awful. Some friends came to visit for awhile, and they suggested Suji needed time away from the scene, time to play with other children. When this was provided for her, she became her old self, and then she was able to spend lovely times with Grandma. Two days before Christmas, Suji went on her own to Grandma's room, held her hand, and read Christmas poems to her.

Grandma died that night. Penelope and her sisters washed and dressed their mother. When Suji woke up in the morning, she asked about Grandma, and was told that her body was still in the room, but she had gone. Did Suji want to go to her? She definitely did, and looked long, and tenderly stroked her arm. Then she went and gathered roses and greens from the holiday bouquets, and arranged them all around Grandma's head and shoulders, very beautifully.

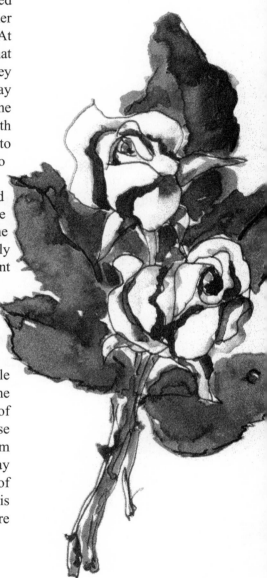

Even when we think someone won't get better, they might be able to get better. Whether it is all-better, or for only a time, that time can make all the difference. It is the privilege and opportunity of those of us who love, to make the space for this to happen. These two mothers and their families showed us that. And, just now I am thinking of another, very special case – someone who today seems to be held to physical existence mostly by the strength of the love of his many caring friends. And yet, every day, his life is full, and a blessing to everyone. Can those of us who are "healthy" always claim that?

When a Friend Is in the Hospital . . .

❧ This is worth repeating: when you go to visit in the hospital bringing quiet optimism, calm and good humor, appreciation for the staff, a willingness to do little comforting things to help, or to just *be* there, that helps the patient. It also helps the nurses and doctors, in many ways.

❧ Nourishing homemade food may be welcome to your friend in the hospital. Hospitals vary in their ability to provide appropriate food, and patients in their capacity to enjoy what is given. What comes from home can be important. See next page for ideas – or, better yet, ask the patient.

Diamond Organics will send a basket of seasonal organically grown fruits anywhere overnight. (Toll-free, 888 674 2642)

❧ Even if you live at a distance, small thoughtful things you send – flowers, books, cartoons, tapes, a basket of fruit – mean so much. Even if you are far away, call. In a long-term situation, sometimes your fresh voice, or a one-time visit, can make a big difference, so even if you are able to help only once, offer.

❧ "Visits were nice but very tiring. JoAnne was wonderful, she'd just talk away in her soothing voice, every word amusing and nothing the least negative. I could just listen and listen."

❧ Your visit helps a convalescent if you are calm and cheerful. If you have reason to think that your presence might cause tension, it would be thoughtful just to send some nice remembrance.

Hospital Food

A friend reports:

"I was in the hospital for eleven days after abdominal surgery. Until the last day, I couldn't eat one thing on the hospital menu. Even a lot of what was brought from home, I couldn't use, or at least not right away; for example, I had asked for fresh orange juice, but it was too acid, and upset my stomach. But every day friends brought some things, and one or two would be just right, and I don't know what I'd have done without that. I know you are thinking I must be a picky eater! Listen to this: my doctor ordered 'non-gas-producing' diet for me, but when my first postsurgical meal arrived, it was a salad consisting of two cups of under-cooked navy beans mixed together with some barely defrosted string beans, all of it drowning in oil and vinegar. Bah.

"Homemade broth, very mild, was what I wanted at the beginning when my digestion was flooey. Barley Tea, too, so soothing! That was the best. Then, lovely homemade applesauce, and rice crackers. The hospital did not offer rice or rice crackers. And yogurt. They provided only teeny four-ounce containers of it, no active culture, with gobs of jam ("fruit") at the bottom. Thank goodness I had plenty from home. The last few days I was there, when I was feeling better, my best treat was one of their packets of cold cereal with some of their jammy yogurt over a bowl of plain homemade yogurt.

"I have never been fond of herb teas, but I did enjoy them at this time."

≥∂

Then again, some people find hospital food just great.

Coming Home

◦ If you are there with the patient when her doctor stops by just before she leaves the hospital, *take notes.* No matter how alert your friend seems, if she has been given pain medication the chances of her remembering anything said at that time are slim indeed. This is the time to find out about diet, activity, bathing, a return checkup appointment, needs for special equipment, medication schedules, anything relevant.

◦ Until she gets her strength back, try to offer her a little juice or food, even a few swallows, as often as she can take it. Real juices like orange or carrot have the most nutrients, but in this case calories are what is most needed so whatever she's willing to take is best.

◦ Any time taking a normal quantity of food seems overwhelming keep appealing tidbits on hand to help a patient eat the needed calories.

NOURISHING SNACKS
juice
muffins
crackers
"good" cookies
hard cheese cubes
dried fruits – raisins, prunes,
    peaches, cranberries
granola or other favorite
    cereal
nuts or nut butter
sandwiches cut in quarters
fresh fruit – strawberries,
    grapes, pieces of melon
halvah

HOT OR COLD
Tofu Bars (page 146)
chocolate milk, smoothie
Thin Soup (pages 113–116)
bite-size vegetables; dip
pudding or custard
frozen yogurt, ice cream
yogurt

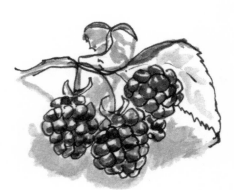

Pills

Coming home from the hospital, it isn't unusual to have many different medications, no two to be taken on the same schedule. Even for someone who's not dopey from pain medication, it's so confusing! Line up all the bottles and gizmos, and make a chart so that it's easy to see what to take when. For capsules, tablets, and pills, the multisectioned pillboxes that pharmacies sell can be wonderfully helpful. Have a notebook to write down each dose as it is taken, for a while at least, especially pain medications. Find out from the doctor what to do if a dose is missed, and what side effects or reactions you need to watch out for.

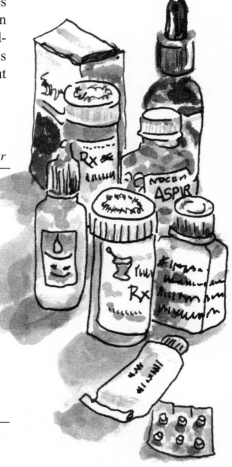

MEDICATION SCHEDULE

	Red pills	Blue pills	Mouthwash	Inhaler
On arising	1			×
At breakfast		2	after	
Midmorning	1			
With lunch		2	after	
Midafternoon	1			×
With dinner		2	after	
Bedtime	2			
As needed				×
Side effects	vertigo		nausea	
Call Dr. at once if:	fainting		vomiting	

When a patient is taking pain meditation, he may not think clearly. Be sure to keep the medication out of reach so that extras won't be taken inadvertently. A grim factoid for you: a study in *The Archives of Internal Medicine* (Oct. 9, 1995) estimates that more than one-quarter of all hospital admissions in the US are the result of prescription-drug misadventures.

Mealtime Suggestions

❧ Eating can seem like a lot of work when you are sick. Calm, upbeat company makes the effort worthwhile. Whether you have much to say or not, sit there with her while she eats. If you feel restless just sitting, have a cup of tea. Avoid distractions like TV, fractious conversation, music.

❧ Say grace together.

❧ In a long illness, it's important to have a predictable daily routine. Keeping mealtimes regular, especially, boosts appetite and digestion. It also puts trail markers in an otherwise amorphous day: the next meal is something to look forward to – or, if meals are difficult, each one becomes an accomplishment for which you can congratulate each other.

❧ The advice about regular scheduling is valuable even if your patient badly needs calories and has a hard time eating enough at meals. When that's a problem, keep nutritious, caloric snacks within reach between meals, for nibbling whenever she feels hungry. In such cases, whatever she might enjoy is the best – choose the most nutritious tidbits you can think of. Some suggestions, two pages back.

❧ Sometimes leafing through a colorful cookbook together will give both of you ideas for foods that would taste good.

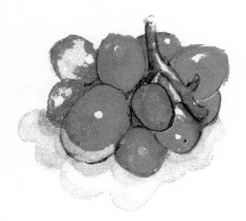

❧ Set a pretty table – cheerful with a bright, colorful tablecloth, napkins, china. On a special day, maybe the setting could be serene and formal. Picnic by the window; dinner by candlelight.

❧ Even a tray can have a tiny bouquet. If you have special china or silverware this might be a time to bring it out.

❧ Cloth napkins, tucked in to protect clothing – not as if she were a baby, but royalty. This can be a little ritual to start the meal. (The napkin for wiping the lips should be extra soft. Paper "dinner napkins" are good for that.)

❧ Serve dessert in a pretty wine glass.

❧ Even if she can't come to the table, can she eat with the family by having her meal nearby, maybe propped up on the couch?

PILLS

❧ If there are pills to take at mealtime, have a little dish that is reserved just for them, perhaps an old-fashioned crystal salt dish, or one of those exquisite Japanese miniature sauce dishes – shallow but with sloped sides, so it is easy to pick up each capsule and tablet. Seeing the special dish is a good reminder for you, and gives the medications their own special, dignified place in the scheme of things.

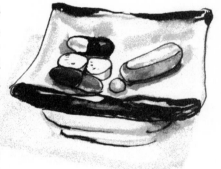

❧ If pills are hard to swallow, often it is easier to take them with food than with liquid. Semisolid savory food is the best of all for this. Children may manage best if the pill is pressed between slices of banana.

❧ Most of us just swallow our pills without giving it a thought. Consider, however: would slowing down, focusing the mind on hoped-for benefits, maybe repeating a short prayer at that time, change our attitude toward "drugs," and open the way for "good medicine" to do its work in the body more harmoniously?

❧ Watch out for generous servings, they can be overwhelming.

❧ Rich aromas, so appetizing at other times, can overwhelm a person whose digestion is off. A patient who will be well enough to join the family for dinner tomorrow may today still find cooking smells nauseating.

❧ If he has a hard time eating enough, avoid serving much liquid before or with meals.

❧ Crunchy, smooth, crispy, cool, warm, spicy, hot, tart, sweet. Contrasts and complements. Favorite chutney, salsa, pickle, and other you-choose condiments can perk appetite, and aid digestion too.

❧ Some medications and some diseases, too, alter taste perception; age can diminish it. Our challenge in the kitchen is figuring out how to compensate – emphasize some tastes, or prepare more highly flavored foods.

Eating is universally recognized as the sign of recovery, renewal, of life. Not for nothing are we caregivers always trying to "get them to eat something." Mostly we are right. Often, though, what would be the biggest help to both our charges and ourselves, is to slow down and really listen to what they think they want. Even if it turns out to be something forbidden or otherwise impossible, you have a clue to how to come up with some alternative that would be OK.

There are times when your patient would agree that he really does *need* to eat, but "I'm not *hun*gry." If you know him well, you will be able to figure out how to help him get past this. Most of us have found if we go ahead and cook the meal, and set it out nicely, then ask him to "just let me show you what I have made – maybe some of it will look good to you," the initial resistance softens, and after a perhaps grudging bite, appetite returns, and he can really enjoy the meal.

Sometimes a bit of sincere advertising can help:

"Of course, you don't want to eat anything. I agree, it is just too much. But, maybe you could take just a bite of this? It is really special, I don't want you to miss it."

"Won't you try just one bite? it isn't too sweet but it is very flavorful. . . ."

"This is made from the recipe Janaki sent from India."

"Look! I have stuffed the tomato the girls brought from their school garden."

"Julia picked this peach only just now, from the tree they planted by the creek when Chris was born. Do you catch the fragrance?"

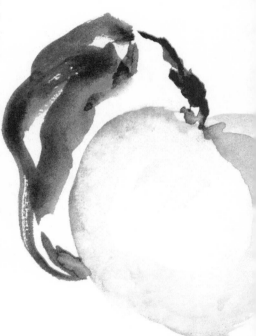

Serving on an Unpredictable Schedule

When you have to hold a meal because your cookee is not hungry yet, the food must be kept cold or hot if it is not going to spoil. Hot, here, means over 140°F, and cold, below 40°F. Remember that anyone who is ill, especially if the immune system is compromised, is less able to defend against even small invasions of bacteria in their food.

Please refer to page 86 for more food safety tips

Simple but elegant Pyrex glass dishes in one- and two-serving sizes have been a wonderful convenience to us. Thick heatproof glass, elegantly simple, with a nice, flat, stable bottom, they move from cold storage to the oven, *bainmarie*, or microwave as needed, and look classy enough to serve in. Their substantial, plain-color lids won't go into the oven, but tolerate hot food inside, from kitchen to table. The thick glass bottom retains a lot of heat, so the food inside doesn't cool quickly.

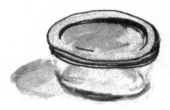

BAINMARIE

One way to keep food hot for serving for as long as an hour is to surround such (heatproof) dishes with an inch of barely simmering water, in a wide skillet over the very lowest heat.

An impromptu, down-home way to serve warm food at bedside: In the kitchen, put a heating pad on your tray, and cover it with layers of clean towel. Plug it in 10 minutes before you expect to serve, to get it good and warm. At serving time, cover the dishes of food (pan lids, for example, to cover plates) and set them on the towel. Top with more towels. Unplug, transport, and then plug in near where your patient will be eating. This isn't as good as a commercial hot tray, but when the meal takes a while, it can make all the difference.

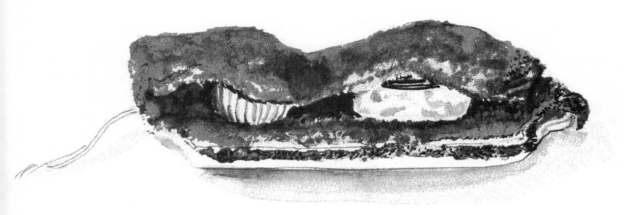

There are days when, well, teamwork it ain't, and the glamour of selfless service pales, perhaps ever so slightly. Maybe, even, your compassion card goes temporarily on the fritz. At times like that, one ploy is to make it a little game to try to get through just this one hour – or just this meal – doing every single thing right.

I remember one particular breakfast. Such attention! Such concentration! Today, surely, I'll claim my very first "Perfect 10." I deftly push back my chair, leaning on the serving spoon handle. St. Patrick's Mousse catapults in a green trajectory Marsward.

Maybe they have openings at NASA?

Spoon-feeding

❧ In the kitchen, cut foods into attractive bite-size pieces before serving time. Break angel-hair pasta, fettucini, or spaghetti into half-inch pieces before cooking, or else chop the cooked noodles before saucing. Cut lettuce and other elements of green salad into thin, short julienne. The effect can be just as pretty, but the salad stays on the fork – requires less chewing too. Thick dressing is easier than vinaigrette.

❧ At mealtime, if things aren't going as smoothly as you would hope, take a minute to put yourself in her place, and try to see what's causing the difficulty. For example, cataracts may make it hard for an older person to see what is happening below the line of vision. There, the solution is trajectory: bring the spoon straight up, and then across horizontally to her mouth, rather than carry it in a straight diagonal line from the plate. That lets her see the approaching mouthful, so she can time the biting accurately. This is a real team effort!

❧ Days of spoon-feeding can give you painful shoulders. This works for (right-handed) me: sitting facing my eater, on her right side with the food far enough inboard that I can keep my elbow on the table while loading up the spoon or fork. Between bites, I make a conscious effort to relax my shoulder completely, even though just for a half-second at a time – the same principle as a mountaineer's "step-rest" that lets a tired climber get all the way to the top.

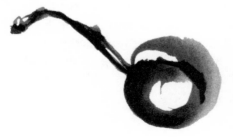

Mouth Care

A nonambulatory patient will feel better if you help him rinse his mouth after eating. Sickness can give a person a stale-tasting mouth, so sometimes it is a comfort to rinse between meals, and maybe even before eating, as well.

Rinsing with a simple salt solution helps keep bacteria down, and promotes healing as well. Mix ¼ teaspoon table salt into a cup of warm water.

If the patient prefers, sometimes a squeeze of lemon or pinch of baking soda may be helpful occasional alternatives to salt. Cool chamomile tea has many beneficial properties in this context. Commercial mouthwashes can be refreshing, also.

Special lemon-glycerine swabs are available from the pharmacy for times when even rinsing is too hard.

❧

Certain illnesses, certain medications and procedures, can predispose a patient to developing a sore mouth. The doctor has effective medications if that happens, but some help can come from the kitchen too.

- ❧ Keep lips soft with lanolin, petroleum jelly, olive oil, swabbed gently on.

- ❧ Rinse as frequently as is comfortable with the salt solution described above.

- ❧ Include yogurt with active cultures in the daily cuisine. Other cultured milk products, and fresh miso, can also help promote a beneficial oral flora.

- ❧ Obviously, when the mouth is sore, we need to cook foods soft, and avoid anything that might be irritating: rough, dry foods; sour, salty, spicy things. In extreme cases, chilled foods and drinks will feel best, and a straw for liquids. When using a straw, the liquid should not be hotter than 120°F, or it can burn the top of the mouth.

- ❧ A bedridden patient whose mouth becomes dry may appreciate commercial artificial saliva, available in squeeze bottle at any pharmacy, and also the lemon-glycerine swabs mentioned above.

RINSING
¼ teaspoon salt
1 cup warm water

TIPS

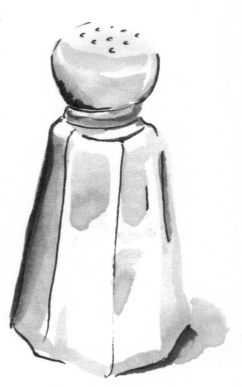

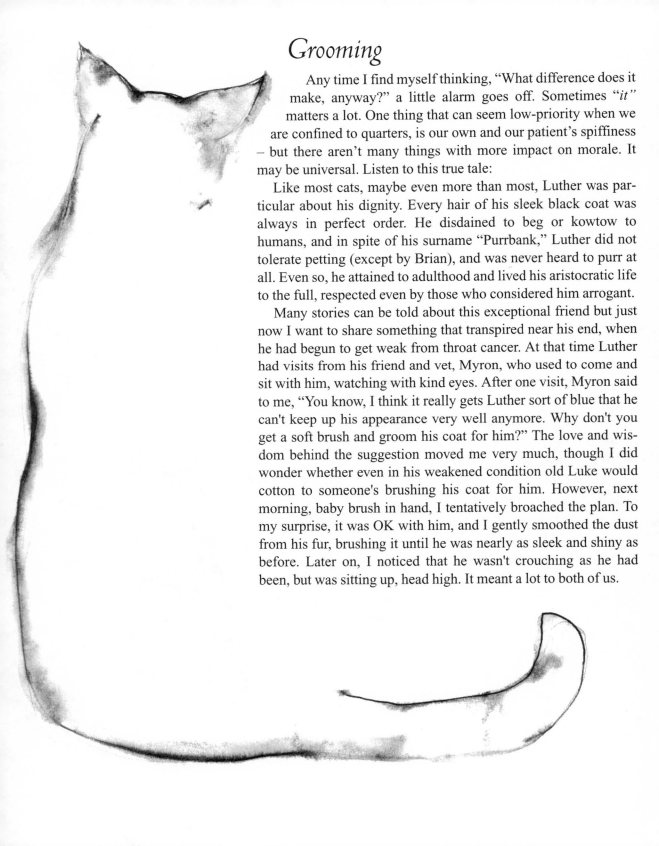

Grooming

Any time I find myself thinking, "What difference does it make, anyway?" a little alarm goes off. Sometimes *"it"* matters a lot. One thing that can seem low-priority when we are confined to quarters, is our own and our patient's spiffiness – but there aren't many things with more impact on morale. It may be universal. Listen to this true tale:

Like most cats, maybe even more than most, Luther was particular about his dignity. Every hair of his sleek black coat was always in perfect order. He disdained to beg or kowtow to humans, and in spite of his surname "Purrbank," Luther did not tolerate petting (except by Brian), and was never heard to purr at all. Even so, he attained to adulthood and lived his aristocratic life to the full, respected even by those who considered him arrogant.

Many stories can be told about this exceptional friend but just now I want to share something that transpired near his end, when he had begun to get weak from throat cancer. At that time Luther had visits from his friend and vet, Myron, who used to come and sit with him, watching with kind eyes. After one visit, Myron said to me, "You know, I think it really gets Luther sort of blue that he can't keep up his appearance very well anymore. Why don't you get a soft brush and groom his coat for him?" The love and wisdom behind the suggestion moved me very much, though I did wonder whether even in his weakened condition old Luke would cotton to someone's brushing his coat for him. However, next morning, baby brush in hand, I tentatively broached the plan. To my surprise, it was OK with him, and I gently smoothed the dust from his fur, brushing it until he was nearly as sleek and shiny as before. Later on, I noticed that he wasn't crouching as he had been, but was sitting up, head high. It meant a lot to both of us.

Getting Better

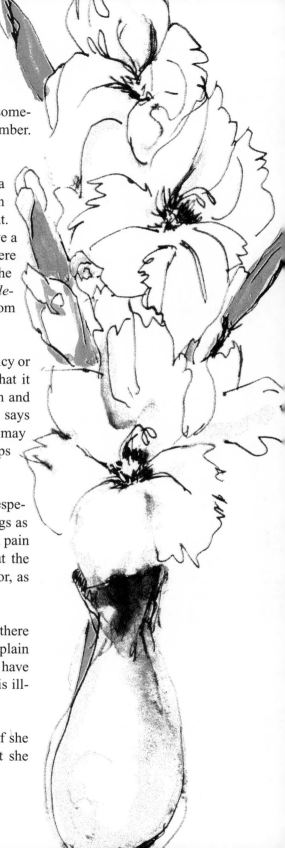

I asked some wonderful caregivers what they would say to someone who was just starting to look after a very ill family member. Maybe you will benefit, as I did, from their responses.

❧ Along with whatever physical distress there may be, a person who is very sick no longer feels in control of his own life, and that in itself creates anguish. *Listen* to your patient. Go out of your way to make sure that every time he can have a say in things, he has it. Of course you would do that when there is a big decision to make. But in a stripped-down life, the smallest things get magnified. *Would you like to have applesauce today, or a banana?* Sometimes there isn't more room for choice than that. Ask.

❧ Remember, when everything is too hot or too cold, too spicy or too bland, too much or too little, nothing, nothing right, that it isn't *you* that's wrong. It isn't *her* fault, either – this is pain and fear speaking. "If you can keep calm and stay pleasant," says Sylvia, "when they are irritable because of their pain, they may not say so just then but they appreciate it so much, and it helps them more than anything you can do."

❧ Even if the illness probably won't be a long one – but especially if it might! – keep a daily journal to record such things as activity, sleep pattern, food, medications, bowel movements, pain level, special problems. You think you will remember, but the days meld into one another, and it is so helpful to the doctor, as well as to you, to have a clear record, both now and later on.

❧ Treat him always with courtesy. Don't let anyone stand there and talk about him as though he's not present. When you explain something, be sure he understands – medical terms may have become familiar to you if you have been studying up on this illness, but they can be scary to the guy on the bed.

❧ Medications can take a tuck in the intellect. Be tactful. If she forgets something, help her save face. Think for her what she might need: adjusting the pillows might be beyond her: *Shall I put a cushion under your knees? Would it help to have your head raised a little?* A bell by the bed, the phone within reach.

❧ No one wants to be unkind. We don't, our patient doesn't. But *we* are not in pain, *we* are not medicated. Who should take the flack? Certain arguments don't have to be won. Certain points don't have to be made. Later on, these memories can haunt you.

HELPFUL BOOKS

A treasure trove of resources: Making Life More Livable: A Practical Guide to Over 1,000 Products and Resources for Living Well in the Mature Years, *by Ellen Lederman (Fireside, 1994).*

Everything but recipes: Keys to Survival for Caregivers, *by Mary K. Kouri (Barron's, 1992).*

In a class by itself, a wonderful book: Share the Care: How to Organize a Group to Care for Someone Who is Seriously Ill, *by Cappy Capossela and Sheila Warnock (Fireside, 1995).*

❧ Performing little services gives the caregiver the chance to show love, says that this is not just a duty. Back rubs, foot massage, hot-water bottle, a careful shave, makeup. Reading out loud. Being there sometimes when you don't have to.

❧ Exercise is so important, it keeps the blood moving around, improves morale, prevents many problems. If it is hard for her to get up and walk, get up and walk with her. If she can only walk around the room, walk around the room every hour on the hour. If she can lift her arms, do pared-down jumping jacks together. Sit for a little in the sunshine. Go for a little drive.

❧ Cleanliness too. There are different sorts of gizmos to help people get in and out of the tub or shower, for example, that can be worth their weight in gold. Check the phone book for medical supply rentals, or look in the *Resources* sections of these books.

❧ Caregivers, look after yourself. Your health and sanity are your most essential tools. Not only your patient, but *you too* need a tasty, healthful diet, fresh air and exercise, comfortable, attractive clothing, a haircut, a manicure. Company, a good laugh. No one can manage this job in isolation. Think about who else could help, and make it possible for them to do it. They will thank you.

And now for some recipes . . .

Thin Soups

The pain in his throat made it hard for him to swallow solid food, so his doctor said to get canned "complete nutrition" liquid. We bought one of each kind, and tried them all. He said they tasted terrible, and it was true. Vanilla flavor diluted by half with double-strength Ginger Tea (page 76), went down easier – but please, couldn't we make something real, something *not sweet?*

We came up with these soups. Simple as they are, and delicious, when we ran the list of ingredients through the computer, they compared favorably with commercial liquid foods.

Our friend recovered on these soups, drinking several ten-ounce glasses a day through a straw. Now he goes for walks on the beach, and enjoys normal meals.

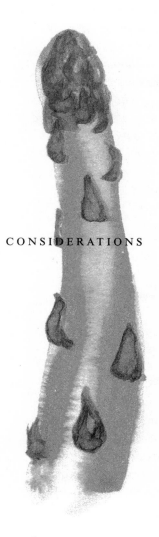

🍠 Vegetables are most nutritious and tasty when fresh, and freshly cooked. However, these soups do keep their flavor in the refrigerator for a couple of days.

🍠 With its concentrated, complete nutrition, convenience, and digestibility, milk is a godsend for caregiver and patient. If yours is lactose intolerant, you can treat milk with lactase enzyme drops, available in pharmacies. Soymilk is certainly also nutritious, but more care is needed to balance its nutrients – a consideration in long-term situations.

🍠 If the need for calories is very great, add small amounts of almond butter or good-quality monounsaturated oil like virgin olive oil to the mixture in the blender. In some special cases, high-fat dairy products like butter or cream cheese can be justified. For most of us who have learned about nutrition for healthy people, this can be hard to accept, but it is true.

🍠 A do-ahead prep we like is to sauté a big chopped onion with several garlic cloves. What a time-saver when cooking for one, to be able to just spoon out a teaspoonful, and perhaps, a clove of garlic. Add them to quicker-cooking vegetables (or juice) to make soup as needed. This turns out to be an elegant procedure anyway because cooked onion keeps its flavor in the refrigerator better than cut raw, and it doesn't stink up the surrounding turf.

If the onion and garlic, or the pepper, pose digestive problems, omit them. If sodium is restricted, leave out the salt. These recipes suited our cookee, and you must suit yours.

Spinach Soup

This quick, delicious soup is thin enough to drink through a straw.

❧

ONE 10-OUNCE CUP

*1 tablespoon chopped onion
   or shallot*
½ small garlic clove
1 teaspoon oil
*¾ cup chopped fresh spin-
   ach, or adjust to taste*
milk to make 10 oz.
salt and pepper to taste

Sauté onion and garlic in oil in a small, heavy pan, cooking until transparent, or else use a teaspoonful you previously prepared. Add spinach and cook, stirring, until soft. Blend smooth using just enough of the milk to cover vegetables in blender. Add rest of milk, salt and pepper.

Depending on the time of year and other factors, the spinach may taste sweeter or more acidic. If the soup seems too strong to you (especially likely when you use skim milk), you may need to reduce the proportion of spinach by blending in more milk, or a little milk powder; or smooth out the flavor by adding some butter or oil, a little nut butter, or a teaspoon of cream, cream cheese, ricotta, or sour cream, depending on your patient's needs.

VARIATIONS

❧ Peas add sweetness; add a spoonful to the spinach as it cooks.

❧ If a thicker soup is acceptable, blend in a spoonful of cooked potato, oatmeal, rice, or pasta. These add beneficial carbohydrates.

For many other variations on this theme, see pages 150–151.

Shallots are single-serving-size onions with terrific flavor – very convenient when cooking for one.

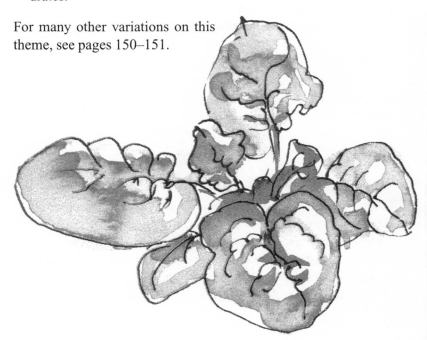

Asparagus Soups

Fresh asparagus juice made in an electric juicer doesn't taste very good, but this soup does. A pound of fresh asparagus, about 16 medium spears, makes about 1½ cups of juice in an electric juicer, and that is what's required for the first recipe. The second recipe uses the vegetable itself, and requires only an ordinary blender.

ॐ

VERY THIN SOUP USING FRESH JUICE

Chop onion and sauté with garlic in oil until golden but not brown – or put previously sautéed onion and garlic in a pan. Add juice, and bring to a boil. Simmer for a couple of minutes. Transfer to blender, cover, and place a folded towel over the top to protect you in case the hot liquid should spew out. Blend smooth, beginning on low speed. Strain. Pour into a quart jar, adding milk to the top, plus salt and pepper.

Serve hot, but at *not more than 120°F for drinking through a straw.*

Three 10-ounce servings.

½ onion
2 cloves garlic
1 tablespoon oil
(or ¼ cup previously sautéed onion & garlic)
1½ cups asparagus juice
milk to make 4 cups
¼ – ½ teaspoon salt, pepper to taste

ॐ

USING CUT ASPARAGUS

Sauté onion and garlic in oil until soft, without browning. Meantime, wash, trim, and chop asparagus, and add to the pan with a couple of tablespoons of water. Cook until tender. Put into the blender with enough of the milk to cover, and blend very smooth. Add milk to fill a quart jar. Season, and heat as needed to serving temperature. This version can usually go through a straw if it is strained.

Three 10-ounce servings.

½ small onion, chopped
1 garlic clove or more, to taste
1 tablespoon olive oil
1 pound (16 medium stalks) asparagus
milk to make 4 cups total
salt and pepper to taste

VARIATIONS

↪ Steam fresh artichokes and use the hearts and leaf-scrapings instead of cut asparagus. Peas are good in this too.

↪ Add ¼ to ½ cup tender green peas to either soup while simmering. Blend and strain, then add the milk.

Red Pepper Soups

Pretty and colorful, very good for variety, and *tasty*. Red peppers are a rich source of carotenes and vitamin C.

❧ Follow the recipe for Spinach Soup two pages back, or the one at the top of page 150, but use chopped, grilled, peeled pepper instead of the fresh chopped raw spinach.

❧ Use any of the pepper purée recipes on page 120, adding broth or milk, as appropriate, to thin to the desired consistency.

&

HOW TO GRILL PEPPERS

Follow one of these three methods to loosen the peels:

❧ *Under the broiler*: Halve the pepper; cut out the stem and veins, remove seeds. Flatten outside-up on a metal pie tin or broiler pan. Broil just long enough to blister the peels, 5 to 10 minutes.

❧ *Oven*: Best way to do several at a time. Put cleaned peppers outside-up on a lightly oiled baking sheet. Place in *preheated* 450°F oven until the peels blister, maybe 25 minutes.

❧ *Directly over a gas burner*: Messy, but fast. Set uncut pepper over the fire, turning with tongs. Allow flame to blister the entire outside. This is not our favorite way because the charred peel is harder to get off.

Once the peel is entirely blistered, use a tong to move the peppers to any pan or bowl. Cover snugly with a plate, lid, or with another bowl. Peppers will steam, which loosens the peels.

When peppers are cool enough to handle, the peel slips off. Discard every bit of the blackened peel, but don't wash the peppers unless you have to, because you lose flavor by doing that.

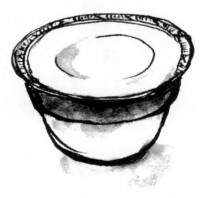

NOTE: Often people tell you to put grilled peppers in a paper or plastic bag. Using a covered dish or pan works much better. Anyway, paper bags are made from recycled paper, and may contain heavy metals or other contaminants. Plastic in contact with hot food leaches harmful chemicals into the food. Who needs it?

Purées

Your patient is getting better, and doesn't need to have everything through a straw – though actual *chewing* is still in the future. Now you can make thicker soups and savory puddings by using less liquid, or by adding a little potato or whole wheat pasta to the blender.

৯৹

Aim for pretty colors and interesting flavors in puréed foods since the texture is a bore.

TIPS

৯৹ The blender and, even more, the food processor, incorporate air into the food, which destroys vitamins and can cause distressing belching. Minimize by chopping foods before blending; blend cold when you can; on low speed, with as little liquid as possible – add the rest of the liquid after blending. *But!* If simply getting enough calories is what's paramount, and if a silky smooth purée is more appealing, blend the purée silky smooth.

৯৹ For the vitamins, minerals, and fiber, thicken purées with cooked whole wheat pasta or brown rice. The flavor of brown rice is sweetly subtle and goes nicely with other foods.

৯৹ Remember there are lots of unblendered foods that patients who need very soft things can enjoy. Some examples: yogurt, timbales (See pages 124–128), cooked vegetables like potatoes and squash, well-cooked pasta, and even beans; tofu, avocado, ripe peaches, bananas and other tropical fruits like mango, cherimoya, and papaya – and, of course, numerous desserts. (It takes a change of mind-set, sometimes, to think of desserts as useful foods, but they can play a helpful role when it is otherwise difficult to get adequate calories and protein. Soft bread (or rice) pudding, cheesecake, custard, of *course* ice cream . . . the list goes on. Much harder to find appealing things that are *not* sweet.)

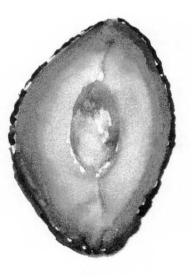

৯৹ Your patient's own favorite solid foods can be puréed of course, and many dishes taste all right that way. The recipes that follow give a range of possibilities using nutritious and versatile vegetables like spinach, asparagus, and red bell peppers.

St. Patrick's Moose

½ – 1 cup cooked spinach
(or half spinach and half
kale), liquid squeezed out
½ cup ricotta cheese, or part
cottage cheese
½ cup nonfat milk, more if
needed to blend smooth
¼ teaspoon salt
black pepper to taste

A *green* dish indeed, unpredictably delicious. Few would ever imagine eating such a thing, but during at least one long convalescence, it was welcome daily fare, and quite a bit got spooned into the cook too. An astonishing aside: the neighbor's visiting toddlers would linger when they knew what was in the blender, not content unless they could have little dishes of it for themselves.

About nutrition we need hardly speak – this is dynamite. By now it won't surprise you to be told that the proportions are variable according to the eater's requirements. The proportion of vegetable can be less (or more); you can add a little grated cheese sometimes, or increase the calories by blending in a teaspoon of olive oil. Later on, when calories are not first priority, gradually reduce the fat, and, finally, substitute cottage cheese for part or all of the ricotta if you have spinach that is fresh and sweet.

Kale is delicious here, and provides the extra nutritional benefits you expect from the cabbage family, but without cabbage's digestive challenge. Kale, incidentally, is a hardy, pretty plant that grows even in the snow. It's so much better when really fresh that we heartily recommend slipping a few seedlings into your fall garden, even a flower garden. Pick only the lowest leaves as you need them, and you'll have kale for nearly a year.

٭

Blend smooth in blender. Using a food processor makes it fluffy, which might be appreciated by some, but the beaten-in air can cause gas for others.

Makes about 2 cups, which is not too much.

Asparagus Purée

In the past few years asparagus has been available year-round. Not exactly seasonal or inexpensive in, say, October – but still, when your cookee needs nourishment, asparagus with its easy digestibility, palatability, versatility, and primo nutrient profile, can be a bargain indeed.

1 pound asparagus, about 16 medium spears
½ onion, chopped
2 teaspoons olive oil/ butter
2 garlic cloves
½ cup buttermilk, to taste
salt and pepper
Parmesan cheese or lemon juice to taste

༄

Wash the asparagus and cut into small pieces. You might choose to set the tips aside to use elsewhere, especially if they are very purple,

Sauté the shallot or onion with the garlic, cooking them gently until the onion is golden/ transparent and the garlic soft. Avoid letting it brown. Add the asparagus and a *little* water; cover and cook until tender.

Put it all in blender with buttermilk, and blend until very smooth. Check seasonings.

Makes about 2½ cups.

FOR SPOON-FEEDING

Delicious as it is. If you want it thicker, blend in a little bit of cooked starchy food like potato or rice, or whole wheat pasta. Or skip the buttermilk, and after blending, fold in 3 tablespoons sour cream.

PASTA

Asparagus Purée makes an incomparable pasta sauce for vermicelli or fettucini. Sauce generously, using a cup of sauce to a cup of noodles. A delicious, very special meal for any occasion, and a nutritious one as well. For gourmet company, cook the asparagus tips with the pasta, or strew them on the top.

SOUP

Blend additional broth or milk into the basic purée to make soup – very good hot or chilled.

TIMBALE

See page 127.

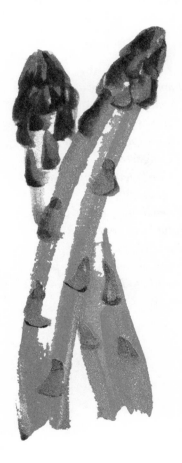

Red Pepper Purée

These mixtures work in many settings as a colorful and tasty sauce or garnish, over or under pasta or vegetables, or spooned around a timbale.

1 large grilled, peeled red
    bell pepper –
    (½ cup chopped)
(1 tablespoon sautéed onion
    and garlic)
water, broth, or milk to blend
salt and pepper to taste

BASIC PEPPER PURÉE

Cut up the peppers and blend smooth in blender, adding sautéed onion and garlic if you want, plus just enough water, milk, or broth to cover the blades. Blend smooth, adding salt and black pepper to taste.

CREAMY PURÉE

Add to basic recipe, 2 or more tablespoons ricotta cheese, sour cream, or cream sauce.

SPICY PURÉE

1 small onion or a shallot,
    chopped
2 cloves of garlic
1 tablespoon minced fresh
    gingerroot
    (or ½ teaspoon powdered
    ginger)
½ teaspoon ground cumin
(pinch cayenne)
2 grilled, peeled red peppers
broth, water, milk, or butter-
    milk to blend

Sauté onion and garlic. When soft, add ginger and spice. Cook until fragrant, just a minute or so, and blend these with the grilled peppers and liquid, and salt and pepper to taste.

With Pasta: For chewing people, red pepper purée is both chic and pretty *underneath* each serving of any small pasta, especially one tossed with colorful, perfectly steamed vegetables: corn kernels, diced green pepper, and peas; or, broccoli florets, cauliflower, and cut green beans. Salt, pepper, maybe a little Parmesan . . .

TENDER PEPPER CROQUETTES

Mix a couple of spoons of pepper purée with a spoonful of ricotta cheese and one of whole wheat bread crumbs. Check salt. Lightly oil a medium-hot griddle and spoon a layer of crumbs on it. Drop the pepper mixture by heaping tablespoonful on the crumbs and flatten slightly to make 2″ disks. When the crumbs brown slightly, sprinkle more crumbs on top of the patties and press down gently. Turn the patties carefully and allow to brown lightly on the other side.

Red Pepper Pasta Pudding

A deep coral-colored savory pudding that was a regular standby for us throughout the purée phase. Whole wheat pasta provides gentle fiber that is most beneficial, and sometimes hard to come by on this kind of diet. Pasta thickens the pudding in a way we found more appealing than thickening by adding whole wheat flour – though that works too; see the second variation, below.

৯

Sauté the onion and garlic in oil. Add the spices and cook about one minute. Put all ingredients in blender, and blend until smooth. Check seasonings. Makes about 2 cups.

VARIATIONS

↬ *Richer and blander:* Omit spices and blend in ⅓ cup ricotta cheese.

↬ *No pasta?* Add 3 tablespoons whole wheat flour to the onion and spices when done, cooking for a minute. Add the milk and cook to a thick sauce, then blend, omitting the pasta. Or use a cooked grain like brown rice instead of the pasta.

↬ *Pasta Unveiled:* When chewing softly is OK, you can make pepper pasta without blending the pasta; in that case, you can double the amount of pasta. For spoon-feeding, whole wheat vermicelli broken into 1″ pieces worked best for us. Incidentally, this dish makes a sophisticated alternative to spaghetti with tomato sauce. Those who need to reduce carbohydrates will find that although, cup for cup, peppers and tomatoes have about the similar amounts of carbohydrate and sugar, peppers make a flavorful, colorful red sauce with half, or even less, vegetable.

2 teaspoons oil
¼ cup chopped onion
1 clove garlic
1 teaspoon fresh ginger
  (or ¼ teaspoon ground,
  or omit)
(¼ teaspoon curry powder)
2 grilled, peeled red bell
  peppers
⅔ cup skim milk
½ cup cooked whole wheat
  pasta
¼ teaspoon salt, and black
  pepper

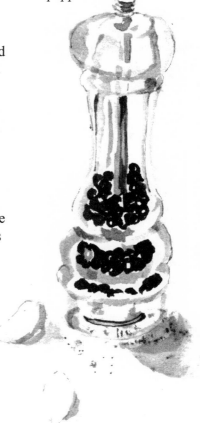

Three Pepper Pasta

a small onion
2 cloves garlic
1 tablespoon olive oil
1" nub gingerroot
½ cup good sherry (or a tea-
spoon of wine vinegar)
1 each, small grilled red,
yellow, and green bell
peppers – about ½ cup
each*
¼ teaspoon salt, and freshly
ground black pepper
1 cup, or more, whole wheat
vermicelli, broken into 1"
pieces

*Instructions for grilling are
on page 116.

A very pretty, lively flavored dish for the next phase, when a little more chewing is OK. Actually, Three Pepper Pasta claims gourmet status. You could serve it proudly to anyone who appreciates good food.

Slice the onion and garlic in thin 1" long slivers, and sauté in oil. Cut the ginger similarly, and add, then add the sherry. Simmer gently while you cut the peppers into similar 1" slivers, then add them to the pan with the salt and plenty of black pepper. Cook the vermicelli, and mix them together. Excellent for spoon-feeding.

VARIATION: Omit the ginger and stir in a tablespoon of grated Parmesan cheese at the end.

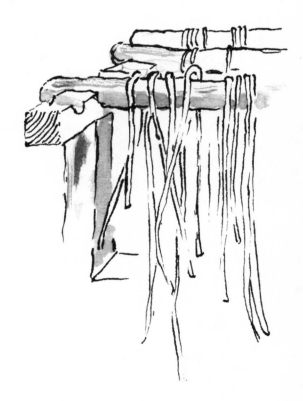

Homemade Pasta

We find whole wheat vermicelli indispensable – easy to spoon-feed, easy to eat, interesting texture for times when chewing other things is too difficult. Cooked whole wheat pasta blended into puréed foods is one way to incorporate beneficial fiber.

Durum flour is the whole-grain version of semolina. It makes noodles with a mellow flavor and golden color that most pasta eaters prefer to the more strident wheatiness of pasta made from ordinary "red" whole wheat flour. You may be able to find whole durum vermicelli ("semolina" is *not* whole grain) in a natural-foods store, but we found it easier to whip out a week's supply with our hand-cranked noodle machine. Here's our current recipe:

3 cups whole durum wheat flour
2 egg whites
½ cup water
½ teaspoon salt

≥∘

Measure the flour into a big bowl. In a separate small bowl, beat the egg and add water and salt, mixing until the salt is dissolved. Make a well in the flour and pour in the liquid, mixing from the center outward until all the flour is included. The dough should be stiffer than bread dough, but not hard as clay. Knead on a floured board until very smooth, cover and set aside to rest for 10 minutes to an hour – or longer in the refrigerator.

Roll thin and cut into strips, by hand or with a pasta machine. Cook some at once and dry the rest on a rack, or spread out on baking sheets to dry. You can store unrolled dough for a few days in the refrigerator.

This dough is suitable for other types of pasta, even ravioli.

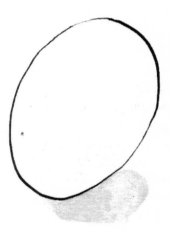

EGGS, NO EGGS

If cholesterol is not a problem and the egg-noodle flavor is enjoyed, you can use 2 whole eggs, or even more, adding the rich nutrients of egg.

We have found it possible, though difficult, to make thin vermicelli without any egg at all. If you omit the egg, be careful not to overcook the noodles.

EGGS, NO EGGS II
Hens in modern egg-producing establishments lead a sad life, and their eggs are not the best, either. Look for eggs from uncaged hens who are not fed slaughterhouse wastes, not given hormones and antibiotics.

Timbales

Timbales *(tam-BALL)* are delicious, elegant, easy to swallow, easy to digest, exceptionally nutritious, and they accommodate themselves to your setting and timing – ideal for caregivers and their charges! *Timbale* means "little drum" – small, savory egg custards, like a tiny quiche without the crust. Historically made with cream and oh-so-rich, you can make them less so, or even fat-free. You can incorporate nearly any vegetable, or no vegetable, or a combination; timbales can be textured, or jello-smooth. Good eating hot, cool, or at room temperature, sauced or plain.

After the first time, they are also exceedingly easy to make, so don't be intimidated by the sea of verbiage that follows – you won't even need to look at it the third time you make them.

Preheat the oven to 325°F. Put a big kettle of water on the fire. Assemble four or so little heatproof dishes, like Pyrex custard dishes, or small fluted molds. Measure them by filling with water so that you will know how much it'll take to fill them up. Dry thoroughly, and grease the insides. Set them side-by-side in a flat baking pan at least as deep as the custard cups.

All your ingredients should be warm-not-hot, though the eggs can be cold. Beat eggs lightly.

When the water boils, turn off the kettle.

Mix the liquids with cheese (and/or other ingredients, if used). Taste, adjust seasoning, then add eggs. Spoon or pour into the custard cups. Set the full cups in their larger pan in the oven and pour hot water around them so that the water comes up to the level of

Liquid: 1½ cups milk, purée, or other liquid
¾ teaspoon salt
⅔ cup cheese, or other flavoring element

2 large or 3 medium eggs

ADJUSTING FLAVOR
Health authorities now caution against ingesting raw egg, so taste the mixture to check the seasoning before mixing in the egg. Make sure the flavor is quite full (plenty of salt) because adding the egg will make it significantly blander.

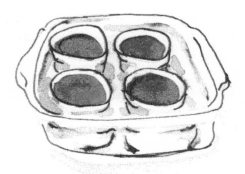

the liquid in the cups. (If your kettle didn't hold enough, it's fine to heat more water, open the oven later, and add more.)

Dot the surfaces with butter if you want to prevent a skin from forming. A light spray of oil works too. If you are planning to unmold the timbales, it won't matter if a skin forms.

Bake until set – 30 to 50 minutes for normal small cups, longer for bigger ones. Exactly how long depends on how your oven holds heat, so it may take you a couple of tries before you know just how long to give them. Here are some clues.

When done:
- they round up on top, and get a slightly golden cast
- they hardly jiggle at all when bumped gently – this gets to be your best clue
- a clean knife inserted 1″ from the center comes out clean
- the inside temperature is 140°F

C A R E F U L L Y remove the big pan from the oven, and use a pancake turner or wide tongs to lift the individual dishes out of the water. *Let them cool for at least 5 to 10 minutes.* Spooning or unmolding them when they are piping hot will cause the timbale to break and weep (maybe the cook, too).

Timbales taste good eaten directly out of their dishes. For more elegant presentation, invert them and remove the cooking dish.

Cool the timbales for 10 minutes. Run a thin sharp knife around the side. Put a small plate upside down over the top and deftly turn both of them over together so that the custard dish sits upside-down on top.

TO UNMOLD

The baking cup should now slip off, leaving the timbale like a quivering hockey puck in the middle of the plate. Sometimes a gentle shake or tap, or tilt, sometimes just a few seconds' wait, helps it happen.

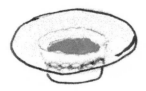  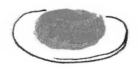

Once the timbale is on the plate, you can spoon a colorful sauce around it, or sprinkle cheese or crumbs or parsley or cilantro on top, or do whatever you think will make it pretty. I have served a timbale as the "filling" inside a big artichoke heart, and have seen them baked in a ring mold, the ring subsequently filled with vegetables. Versatile, indeed! Catastrophes can be stirred, and eaten from the cup. The first timbale I ever saw was a very large one made by Julia Child. When she unmolded it, it split down the middle, with five million people watching. She didn't get flustered at all; she just spooned some veggies into the cleft, added sauce, and commented that most people wouldn't even know the diff.

TAILORING TO SUIT   In its simplest form a timbale is made of milk, cheese, and egg (salt, pepper, nutmeg). The rule is half a cup of egg (two large or three medium eggs), or four yolks or whites, to set $1\frac{1}{2} - 2$ cups of milk, or other liquid. Including more egg makes a sturdier timbale; for your first adventure, you could use four eggs to $1\frac{1}{2}$ cups of milk. Use $\frac{3}{4}$ teaspoon salt for these amounts, or $\frac{1}{2}$ teaspoon with a substantial amount of cheese. Some vigorous flavoring element like cheese *is necessary* because cooked by themselves plain egg and milk are horrid.

↜ *Reduce the fat:* Use low-fat or skim milk, or puréed vegetables for the liquid, substituting part of the egg yolk with white; moderate the cheese content.

↜ *No fat*: Combine a *flavorful* vegetable purée with lightly beaten egg whites. While planning such a dish, remember that in addition to helping hold the custard together, egg yolks increase tenderness and add flavor. When you leave them out you need more seasoning and more care in the baking – be sure to have the surrounding water up to the level of the custard, and don't let the oven temperature get above 325°F, or the timbales will be tough.

Spinach Timbale

Blend the spinach, half the milk, and the cheese. Add the rest of the milk, and salt and pepper to taste, overseasoning slightly to compensate for the egg. Check seasoning. Beat the egg slightly and add it, then pour into cups and bake as described in the last 3 pages.

Spinach Timbale has a charming tendency to layer as it bakes so that the top (bottom, if unmolded) is very green and the bottom (top) creamy pale yellow, with delicately layered shades in-between. If you underdo the cheese, that creamy top part can be pretty awful.

Makes 2 servings.

½ cup chopped, cooked spinach, water squeezed out
1 cup milk
½ cup grated dry jack, Parmesan, Gruyère, or other flavorful cheese
¼ teaspoon salt, and pepper
2 eggs or 3 whites

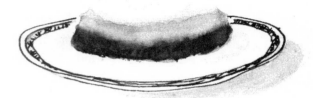

Asparagus Timbale

Combine ingredients and pour into custard cups, baking according to the directions in the last 3 pages.

Makes 3 cups.

One recipe asparagus purée, page 119
3 lightly beaten eggs
3 tablespoons grated Parmesan cheese
½ teaspoon salt
black pepper

VARIATIONS:

↬ Add half a cup of tiny peas, and/or two tablespoons of chopped coriander leaves, before or after blending.

↬ Substitute freshly cooked artichoke hearts and scrapings for the asparagus. Yum.

↬ *Low fat:* Omit the cheese and add 2 teaspoons lemon zest plus a little lemon juice to taste; use 5 egg whites instead of the whole eggs.

↬ *Quiche:* Asparagus Timbale mixture makes an incomparable quiche filling. The quantities given are about right for an 8″ pie pan or the equivalent. Arrange sautéed tips on top for extra flair.

Timbale Manifestations

Timbales are so nutritious and so easy to eat, they can become a standby, especially for feeding someone who is quite frail. Having a repertoire of interesting variations keeps meals (and the cook) from getting dull. Using vegetable purées adds color, and helps balance meals nutritionally too.

Blend the following smooth with milk or soymilk as required. Season to taste with salt and pepper. Strain if a smooth timbale is wanted:

⊹ Freshly cooked artichoke heart and leaf scrapings, with optional sautéed onion, garlic, peas. Parmesan cheese.

⊹ Simmer corn with onion, bell pepper, chili powder, and garlic – a flavorful purée with or without a dose of cheddar.

⊹ All the Red Pepper Purées (page 120) make luscious timbales, most successful when egg yolks are included.

OTHER IDEAS FOR SERVING TIMBALES

Bake one layer of one color and then carefully spoon on a second color and bake that.

For fun for chewing eaters, distribute in custard cups before pouring in the liquid, lightly cooked, *well drained*:

⊹ Chopped spinach (and tiny peas, plus grated Parmesan or dry jack cheese, or Gruyère)

⊹ Broccoli florets (and cheddar or Gruyère)

⊹ Asparagus pieces (and Parmesan or Gruyère)

⊹ Sautéed mushrooms

⊹ Colorful mixture of diced vegetables

. . . or, how about dessert?

Cup Custard

Most soothing, digestible, and nourishing of desserts – easy to eat when nothing else will go down. Very easy to make, also, once you have your system together.

❧

Preheat oven to 325°F. Set 2 quarts or so of water to boil.

Gather together: Pyrex custard cups or ceramic coffee mugs, (or a bowl or baking dish) with total capacity measuring 3 cups, plus another deep flat baking dish all of them fit into. Mix all the ingredients and pour into cups. Dust the tops with nutmeg if you like, and tiny dots of butter. Set the cups in the baking pan and put that in the oven. Carefully pour hot water around the cups so that it comes up as high as the liquid in the cups, near as possible.

Bake until the custard is set, about 40 minutes, depending on the size of the containers – bigger containers take longer. Check doneness by inserting a clean knife into the custard an inch from the center; if it comes out clean, it's done. Remove, and cool. Store covered in the refrigerator.

2 cups milk, warm but not hot
2 large or 3 medium eggs, lightly beaten
⅓ cup light honey, or light brown sugar
pinch salt
½ teaspoon vanilla

(nutmeg)
(dots of butter)

For many tips on making custard, turn back a few pages to the directions for making Timbales. They are savory custards really, and their longer instructions contain many helpful details.

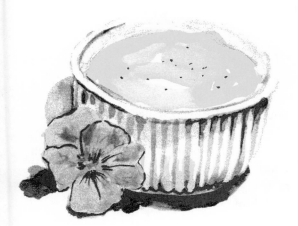

Aspics

A fun change of pace for someone who is not chewing, or for a child. Savory vegetarian "Jello" set with agar-agar can provide a matrix for any fruit or vegetable, and be molded into tempting shapes.

Tiny star and flower molds provide easy forms, but if none of these lurk in your cupboard, make aspic in little custard cups or else in small square containers like sandwich boxes. Once it has set, you can cut it into cubes or turn it onto a board and use cookie cutters, or your imagination, to get desired shapes.

Some fans could eat nearly any amount of this stuff, but for most people, just a little spot for color and zest is adequate to the task. Garnish with chopped parsley or cilantro or other herb, or with a little dab of sour cream or some other cool sauce (or purée) for contrasting color.

TIPS

꙳ Choose intensely flavorful purées to mask the seaweed nuance that reveals agar's antecedents to any alert palate.

꙳ Have ready the molds you want to use. Measure them with water to be sure of the amount of liquid you will need, then dry them well and grease them by *rubbing* the inside generously with a lecithin spray or mixture. (See margin, next page.)

꙳ To make a smoother, mellower, more custard-like aspic, without changing the setting strength of the agar or reducing its clarity, aficionados add a teaspoon of kuzu powder per cup, stirring that into the cool purée before adding it to the simmering agar broth. Bring the mixture back to the boil long enough to clear the kuzu.

꙳ You can dissolve the agar in any liquid, but if it isn't a clear one, you may find it hard to tell when the agar is completely dissolved, *and that is ee-sen-tial.* Usually the package says it takes about 3 minutes, but it may take 10, even, depending on the agar.

꙳ Note that agar sets at 90°F so a purée can't be *ice* cold when you add it to the simmering broth, or the agar will set in horrid lumps before it gets mixed, and you will have to heat it and simmer it all over again to de-lump.

Savory Aspic

Choose any of the purées on pages 117–120, or a flavorful tomato sauce, or a commercial juice like "Spicy-hot V-8." Simmer the agar in broth (or water) until it is completely dissolved.

Stir in the room-temperature purée or sauce or juice, mix well, and pour into mold(s).

You can make it set faster by placing the molds in ice water, or in the refrigerator, but anyhow it only needs to cool to 90°F, so it is much faster and sturdier than animal gelatin, which has to be really cold to set.

TO UNMOLD, heat the outside of the mold slightly – metal molds can be put on the gas burner *briefly!* If yours is a plastic or glass container, make sure the aspic is very firm, then dip the outside of the container in very hot water long enough to heat the container but not the contents. Loosening the sides with a knife or toothpick is fair, and generally necessary, if the mold is not made of metal. Put a plate over the top of the mold, invert both, and tap gently so that the aspic slips out. This is the tricky part, and why the lecithin is necessary. Don't panic, it will almost always come out, but if worse comes to worst, reach for the melon baller . . .

Because it sets when it reaches 90°F, you can serve it either at room temperature or cold.

1 cup of broth
2 tablespoons agar-agar
1 cup flavorful purée

Check package directions! Normally, 1 tablespoon agar + 1 cup of liquid gives a set that is firm but not cement-like.

1 tablespoon flakes
 =1 teaspoon powder

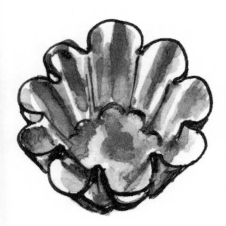

GREASE
Canned lecithin sprays like Pam are ubiquitous and convenient. Here's an effective, inexpensive homemade equivalent that delivers even less fat:
Blend ½ cup cooking oil with 2 tablespoons liquid lecithin. Store in the refrigerator. Spread THIN *to grease anything.*

Sweet Vegetarian "Gell-o"

¼ cup agar-agar flakes
4 cups sweet fruit juice,
  preferably flavorful and
  red

Optional:
2–4 cups bite-size fresh
  sweet fruit: peeled ripe
  peaches, bananas,
  grapes, strawberries
  – soft fruits, if chewing is
  difficult

We think the tapioca version on page 47 tastes better, but if you are after a firm Jello-like effect, here's the vegetarian option. Since it is made with real fruit juice instead of food coloring and sugar, the flavor is more interesting, but the result is admittedly not quite so glassily transparent. You also don't get colors like grass green and taxicab yellow, though the cranberry, raspberry, strawberry, grape, blue- and blackberry juice versions produce beautiful results. Varietal white grape juice makes an amber-colored gel with splendid flavor, especially nice with chunks of fruit. Don't try orange juice, as it is far too sour, and its opacity is off-putting.

For tips about agar, please turn back a page.

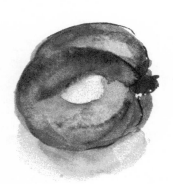

جٻ

Mix agar and juice, and simmer gently until the agar is completely dissolved, with no visible trace of it left at all. Pour into an 8″ × 8″ pan, or warmed-up clear glasses, or Jell-O, or whatever you like. Let cool to about 100F° (just 15 minutes or so), then gently stir in fruit, and refrigerate until ready to serve.

VARIATIONS

↝ Nutritious and surprisingly tasty: mix part with an equal amount of cottage cheese for the glop they knew and, perhaps, loved in the days of yore.

↝ Do check out the tapioca version on page 47. Similarly simmering dried fruit like cranberries, apricots, peaches, nectarines, white raisins, and cherries along with the agar and juice mixture in the above recipe works fine when your patient is up to the somewhat more challenging chewing and digesting these tasty fruits require.

New Life, New Lifestyle?

A few words here for the caregiver and patient who have received a mandate for making a major change in eating patterns.

Maybe you cook for the patient, maybe you have for years and years. You know all too well what likes and dislikes are in place – the prospect of reversing them may seem daunting. But the potential rewards are great, for both of you.

Teamwork is the key. Cook and eater face the challenge hand-in-hand. You know each other so well – choose the right moment, talk it over. Can you both agree that you want to live a long time together, feeling great? Can you agree that eating differently, exercising, will contribute to that? Then agree to set out on this new adventure, determined to make it work, and to make it fun, each for the other. Shake on it.

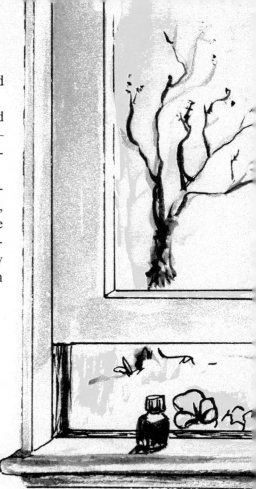

SOME SUGGESTIONS

↬ Sit down together and think about your meals as they have been. Are there some things you hardly need to change? What can you change effortlessly? For example, if a cup of soup, bagel, and fresh fruit sound good, you've solved lunch.

↬ Often it's easier to substitute something else, than diminish a favorite. For example, if butter is now forbidden, it may work better to substitute hot cereal for awhile, than to try to eat dry toast at breakfast.

↬ Keep in mind that the palate can be educated, and tastes do change. Meat-and-potatoes people who stick with a fat-free diet are amazed to see their liking for greasy stuff gradually fade away. At first, for sure, they just enjoy how good they feel. But after awhile, they come to relish the food itself, and can't imagine eating those former favorites.

Other helpful ideas about eating a new way, page 30.

↬ Be daring about trying new foods. If one experiment is a disaster, laugh about it together and try another. Keep a record.

↬ Most people do better with real foods rather than synthetic imitations. Studies have shown that people who go on no-fat diets lose their taste for fat. Those on similar no-fat diets, but with imitation fat included, do not. The same applies to sugar. Nonetheless, "fakes" may help ease transitions for non-swashbucklers.

- When family and friends invite you over, be matter-of-fact about the new regime. If they want to cook for you, let them know that relaxing the diet is not an option. Tell them why. They may be glad to follow your guidelines. If not, go there *after* dinner. *No blame.*

- Study up. Go to the bookstore, health education center, library. Talk with your doctor, dietitian, librarian. Seek out information, motivation, recipes. The more you know, the more possible it will seem, and the more your enthusiasm will grow.

If you are the cook, you probably have specialties. Maybe you have been famous for your Bavarian Cream Chantilly. It *is* dismaying to think that Never Again will you hear the oohs and aahs as you set it out at special birthday dinners. Still, put that recipe aside. Now is the time to come up with new specialties, find new favorites. Things won't ever be the same, but they can be better.

Taking on this challenge as an adventure together can be unexpectedly wonderful for both of you. For sure, it is worlds more fun than facing it like a prison sentence. Cultivate your sense of humor. Always keep high expectations for each other, and whatever slips there may be, don't give up on the other person at all. If mealtime seems bleak during the transition period, shower your love in every other way you can think of. Food isn't everything.

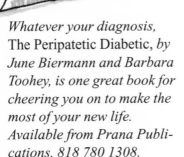

Whatever your diagnosis, The Peripatetic Diabetic, *by June Biermann and Barbara Toohey, is one great book for cheering you on to make the most of your new life. Available from Prana Publications, 818 780 1308.*

If you are a dedicated gourmet who needs to say goodbye to fat, Dean Ornish's excellent cookbooks will be just your cup of tea.

John and Mary McDougall's books offer many fat-free recipes, and fearsome motivations.

Neal Barnard's Eat Right, Live Longer *(Harmony Books, 1995) is so positive and encouraging that you can hardly believe you ever wanted to eat the old way.*

Caregivers' Corner

This chapter is a bouquet of things to make life better for you, the caregivers. These are the recipes we have leaned on during our own caregiving experience over the past several years. One or another of them may be useful to you as well.

The Basics

When Mom landed in the hospital, we discovered that Daddy was pretty much at sea in the kitchen. The following survival techniques grew out of what his daughters sent along to him. If you are an old hand in the kitchen, you can skip over the following few pages.

To start with, here are five easy checks to be sure you get what your body needs for good health every day:

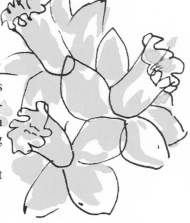

❧ *Detour around junk food*, which includes anything fried. Minimize heavy fat like thick salad dressings, mayo, butter, bakery stuff; yeah, and meat.

❧ *Get 4 servings of whole grain foods* – a serving is only 1 slice of bread, ½ cup pasta or brown rice, so that's easy. White-flour products have had their nutrients removed, and don't count.

❧ *Have 3 servings of vegetables*, including at least 1 dark green one. (Serving size here is nearer to a cup – 2 cups for salad.)

❧ Plus, some beans, or a cup of milk or yogurt.

❧ Fruit, some time in the day.

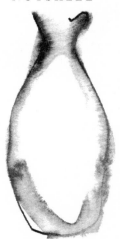

❧ Beyond that, eat a variety of nutritious foods, enough to maintain your weight where you want it. And – get some exercise! That's what moves the blood around, nourishing the cells and taking out the garbage.

If you don't take animal products, please include a vitamin B-1 2 supplement in your regime.

BREAD

That most basic standby for toast and sandwiches really can be a "staff of life." Take time to find a *100% whole wheat* bread you thoroughly enjoy. Check the label; if it isn't "100% whole" then it is refined flour, a "staff" that won't support anyone.

Keep sliced bread in the refrigerator if you won't eat it within a few days, or in the freezer for sandwiches or toast.

Some housebound caregivers tell us they find baking their own bread wonderfully therapeutic. If you think you might like to try, we modestly recommend *The Laurel's Kitchen Bread Book*. Besides lucid instructions, it has a great section on fitting baking into any kind of schedule.

Some automatic bread machines can make whole wheat bread. Others destroy whole wheat dough during an overlong second kneading period, and turn out bricks. Friends with such machines still find them useful for preparing pizza dough or cinnamon rolls – they just remove the dough after the first rise, before the second kneading.

VEGETABLE SOUP

In a big heavy-bottomed soup pot, sauté a chopped onion until golden, adding garlic and some chopped celery or green pepper, if you like. Add stock or water and bring to a boil. Stir in whatever vegetables are in season, chopped attractively – start with slower-cooking ones like potatoes, carrots, and green beans, and end with delicate greens like spinach or parsley and fresh herbs.

Leftover grains, beans, or noodles are welcome and contribute substance to the pot; so does tomato sauce or almost any other leftover sauce. Add tomato in any form after the veggies are tender so their colors stay bright. Milk-containing sauces burn easily, so add them at the end also.

If you want a thick, stewey soup and have no sauce, put part of the cooked soup into the blender and blend smooth, returning the purée to the pot. This simple soup is a perfect way to use up all sorts of valuable little odds and ends.

Vegetables are important for keeping your health at its best. Fresh is ideal, frozen almost as nutritious, though not so delectable. One quick and easy way to prepare fresh vegetables is to steam them. If you use a steamer basket, it's virtually foolproof.

Different veggies take different times to get done – mostly, the harder and bigger they are the more time they take. For instance, carrots and potatoes in big chunks take the longest, about 20 minutes, green beans take 10, spinach, less than a minute. You can judge the quantities, but remember that the softer, wetter veggies cook down into smaller amounts, zucchini to one-third, and spinach more, to about an eighth, so a quart of raw spinach leaves make half a cup cooked, depending on how packed the quart was, of course. You'll get the hang of it so fast, don't worry.

Here we go. If you have a steamer basket, set it in a pot whose lid will fit tight over the steamer when it is piled with whatever you plan to cook. Boil an inch of water in the pan, set the steamer in place, put the vegetables in the steamer, cover tightly, turn the heat to low, and simmer until tender.

The smaller you cut, the quicker they cook, so by slicing carrots thin and zucchini thicker, for example, you can do them in the same time.

A heavy pan will keep things warm, and even continue to cook for a while, after the fire is out.

If you don't have a steamer, then a heavy pan, or one "clad" with a copper or aluminum layer on the bottom, will conduct heat well enough to cook vegetables without a steamer basket insert. Do everything just the same except use less water, stir a couple of times, and keep an eye and ear alert to prevent scorching.

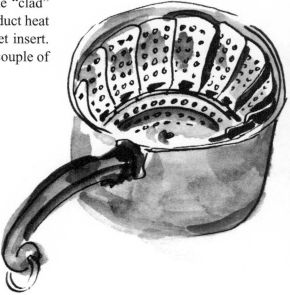

STIR-FRY

Sauté means to cook over high heat in only a little oil, stirring all the while.

Quick and tasty. Gather your fresh vegetables, wash and cut them bite size. Or, cut them up as you cook, like this: put a little oil in the bottom of a wok or a big heavy skillet, and heat it while you cut up a small onion. Put the onion in and stir, then reduce the heat and add a garlic clove. Let them cook over medium heat while you cut a big handful of green beans bite size. Stir it in. Add a couple of spoonfuls of water if the beans start to stick; stir often. Quarter a tomato or two, and maybe slice a small yellow zucchini and add them, stirring, not rushing. Cover the pan. While it simmers, chop a bunch of spinach and when the tomato shows signs of softening, stir in the spinach. A handful of freshly chopped basil, if you have some. Add salt and pepper, and you're ready for the pasta, or rice. (For a warm, subtle garlic flavor, remove and discard the clove after the vegetables have cooked; to get more of the taste, crush the cooked garlic with a fork and return it to the pan.)

For an ambiance that is more Oriental than Italian, leave out the tomato, and use bok choy instead of spinach. Include chunks of broccoli, sliced carrot, whole snow peas, even peeled, sliced, fresh water chestnuts, why not! A tablespoon of soy sauce mixed with a tablespoon of sherry (or rice vinegar, or water) plus ½ teaspoon cornstarch stirred smooth, goes in near the end, when the vegetables are crunchy-tender. If you like the nip, add a tablespoon of minced gingerroot, too. Toss to coat everything. Put the lid on, and let stand a minute to be sure the cornstarch cooks. Top with toasted sesame seeds; serve on rice.

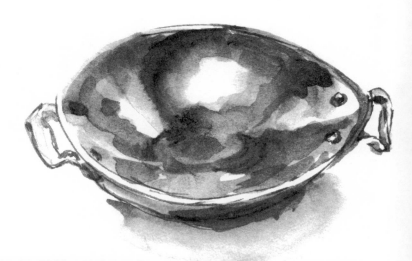

Use a big pan, say, 3 quarts minimum. Fill it about two-thirds full of hot water and bring that to a boil. Add a teaspoon of salt, which makes it boil harder. Put in the pasta and cook until it seems done to you. Whole wheat takes longer to cook than white – 20 minutes for spaghetti, the longest, but worth it.

Put a colander in the sink and pour the boiled pasta and water into it. Return the drained pasta to the pan, and stir in the sauce. Serve right away, while it's hot. If there has to be a wait between cooking and saucing, stir in a few drops of olive oil to keep the pasta from sticking together.

¼ pound
  = 2 cups cooked
feeds 2 generously
needs ½ cup sauce, about

🌤 Put your stir-fry on top, or mix it into the pasta. Good with rice too.

SIMPLE SAUCING

🌤 Drop a handful of frozen peas, maybe some cut-up asparagus, into the noodles 5 minutes before the end of cooking. Drain and toss with black pepper, a little olive oil. Fresh parsley or basil, maybe some Parmesan cheese.

🌤 When you put the water on to boil for the pasta, cut up an onion and sauté it, adding some garlic cloves if you want. Then a couple of cut-up tomatoes, just to soften through. (A bit of sherry, some olives, maybe broccoli chunks or artichoke hearts, could go here too.) Toss with the hot pasta and add a little Parmesan and/or parsley or basil. Black pepper. (Remember to crush the garlic.)

🌤 There are some excellent sauces in jars on the supermarket shelf, even some with organic tomatoes, and no-fat, or low-fat options. They tell how much to use on the jar. Best if the pasta and sauce both be hot, but rules are made to be bent.

RICE   For stovetop rice for the two of you, boil 2 cups of water in a heavy pan. Add ¼ teaspoon salt. Add 1 cup of rice and let the water return to the boil. For brown rice, which is far more nutritious and flavorful but doesn't always come with instructions, boil 5 minutes, then reduce heat to *minimum,* and cook till the water is all absorbed, about 45 minutes. Make sure the heat is very gentle for the last part of the cooking. Someone once wrote me that this was his biggest cooking challenge. He finally solved it by setting one burner rack on top of another, and the pot on that! It works.

TROUBLESHOOTING: At the end, if the rice is slushy, uncover the pan and heat gently to cook the water out. (If there is really a lot of water, you may have measured wrong. Strain off the water and let the rice stand covered for 5 minutes or so.) Or, on the other hand, if the rice seems hard and chewy, add 2 tablespoons more boiling water, cover, and let it have 10 more minutes. It's rare to get it just right the first time because so much depends on the heft and shape of the pan, and how much steam can escape. But soon it'll be second nature, so easy. As the Chinese mother traditionally wishes her new daughter-in-law, "May your rice never be gummy."

OTHER GRAINS COOK EVEN QUICKER
Cook in the same fashion (exceptions noted):

- *Bulgur wheat*, 15 minutes
- *Couscous*, 10 minutes
- *Buckwheat*, 15 minutes
- *Quinoa*, 20 minutes. Wash quinoa well in a fine-mesh strainer before you cook it. It has a natural insecticide on it that's bitter.
- *Polenta*, 25 minutes – less if the grind is fine. Mix the corn with an equal amount of cold water, then stir in 3 measures of boiling water. Stir continuously or, better, cook in a double boiler.

And – don't forget baked potatoes! See page 36.

Beans are easy to eat, delicious, low in fat, a nutritional gold mine. Also cheap. Dry beans cook effortlessly in an electric slow-cooker ("crockpot") – they keep their flavor, shape, and color beautifully.

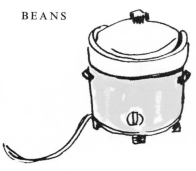

If cooking beans from scratch seems overwhelming, canned beans are still a bargain. Check the label to make sure they don't have fat added, and try to find the brand with the least salt (sodium). Some canned beans are so salty they make you choke – if you get that kind, rinse them off in a strainer.

BEANS DON'T HAVE TO GIVE YOU GAS

The night before, sort through the beans, chucking out dirt, rocks, moldy and damaged ones. Rinse the good ones thoroughly with hot water, and set them to soak in double their measure of boiling water. Next evening, rinse them well again, and put into the crock pot with new boiling water. Cover and let them cook overnight on low, with a towel on top of the crock to conserve heat. They'll be ready for breakfast. *Breakfast?!* Well, of course. Or lunch, or whatever. Freeze the extras in nonmetal ice cube tray for squares to add to Minestrone.

If you don't have a crockpot, cook the soaked beans on the stove. Start with plenty of water. Once boiling, reduce the heat until the beans dance lazily in the pan. You can cover them loosely but they'll boil over if the lid slips down and gets tight. Check and stir from time to time and add water if they are getting dry. Beans take different amounts of time to cook on the stove, from split peas and lentils, at about half an hour, to kidneys and limas, closer to an hour, to navy, pinto, and soy, 3 hours or so. Adding salt, onion, oil, or anything else increases beans' cooking time.

You don't really *have* to soak them beforehand but it does go a long way to preventing them from causing gas, and they take about ¾ as long to cook.

Long ago I learned to make real French Omelettes from a slender volume written by a Parisian woman who operated a tiny omelette shop around the corner from a theatre in London, where her famous omelettes sold like hotcakes after every performance. In these days of Low-Fatness, I hardly ever get to make omelettes any more. An exception comes when someone is convalescing, when there's a place for "building" foods; and caregivers, too, occasionally need something quick and nutritious.

I made omelettes for my mom after she got out of the hospital, using just one egg. Two eggs is normal, three is maybe top limit for flipping. (No need to flip.) Also you can use 2 whites and 1 yolk if you want "lite," but cook on lower heat because whites get tough if they cook too hard.

Break the egg in a bowl and add a pinch of salt and some pepper, and about ½ teaspoon water per egg. Yes, water! It makes the omelette light. Beat with a fork, about 17 beats.

Meantime, heat your pan over a medium-hot flame. Test for hotness by dripping one drop of egg in the pan. It should cook at once, but not burn immediately. When ready, put a little butter in the pan. With a nonstick skillet, you don't need any butter; maybe just barely touch the pan with the butter stick, for flavor.

A good omelette pan is like a crepe pan, see page 32.

Pour the egg into the pan and turn the pan to spread the mixture over the bottom. Lift the egg with the fork, while with your other hand you tip the pan to let the raw part run underneath the cooked part. (Use a nonmetal implement with a nonstick pan.) When the surface of the egg doesn't run any more, turn off the fire. Flip, or gently fold, half the omelette over the other half, making a semicircle. For larger omelettes, fold both sides over the middle.

If you want to put cheese, or salsa, or jam, or whatever, inside, you can spoon it on one half before you do the folding, and you can add a topping, too, like a sprinkle of parsley or Parmesan cheese. Cover the pan with the serving plate and let it stand for a minute or so. That heats the plate and gently finishes the cooking, so that the egg isn't at all raw, but not tough from overcooking either, and the omelette is just warm enough to eat.

If you choose a filling that needs to be cooked – onions or tomatoes, for example – cook them in the pan before the egg, then pour the egg over them, following the directions above just the same, lifting the cooked filling so that the liquid egg flows under it. When you fold the omelette, the filling will be on the inside.

Granola

Easy and satisfying. We make it once a week nowadays, usually the plain version, maybe with raisins. Good even without oil, because it's so fresh, but even a small amount of oil improves crunchiness quite a lot.

৯৯

Preheat the oven to 325°F.

Put the rolled oats in a big bowl.

Mix the liquids with the sugar, spice, if used, and salt. Stir quickly into the oats – until they are moist, but not until they begin to clump.

Spread on cookie sheets, then put into oven promptly. Bake only until evenly golden. This may take as much as an hour.

Stir in the fruit and nuts, wheat germ or bran, then cool completely before storing airtight.

Makes 9½ cups, without any of the optional ingredients.

৯৯

PREPARATION NOTES

↬ For this amount, you will need 2 12″ x 18″ baking pans with sides. If you're using only 1, mix half a recipe at a time because when the mixture has to wait between mixing and baking, the granola gets clumpy and doesn't bake evenly. Underbaked clumps stale swiftly.

↬ Choose rolled oats according to how much you like to chew: Old Fashioned thick oats have a lot of character – they can be tough – especially if you don't use any oil. "Thin," a.k.a. Quick, or medium oats are tenderer, but can lack substance. Including oil gives any kind of oat both tenderness and crunch (and fat calories, alas.)

↬ Some friends like the oats plain and untoasted, with raisins and nuts – classic *muesli*. Since oats are steamed in order to roll them, they *are* cooked. But they are *very dry*. Never eat a lot at one time without plenty of liquid.

↬ If you mean to store your supply for more than a few days, leave raisins and other fruit to add later. Their water content accelerates staling.

2 quarts rolled oats
¾ cup apple juice
or water(plus the zest
of 1 lemon)
½ – 1 cup brown sugar
½ teaspoon salt

OPTIONAL GOODIES
¼ – ½ cup oil
1 teaspoon cinnamon
or ¼ teaspoon cardamom
or 1 teaspoon fennel seeds,
or ground fennel
½ cup raisins
or other dried fruit
½ cup toasted sunflower
seeds,or chopped,
toasted nuts
¼ – ½ cup toasted wheat
germ and/or wheat bran

Stewed Prunes

Much beloved for topping breakfast cereal or yogurt, and justifiably respected as a gentle, effective laxative, good old stewed prunes are finding a chic new role as a fat replacer in baked goods (see pages 51 and 54). Simplicity itself to make.

Rinse whole dried prunes and put them in a pot. Cover with water and bring to a boil, then lower heat and simmer until the prunes are soft and puffy – usually about half an hour, depending on the prunes. Let cool, and store in the refrigerator. For extra flavor, tuck slices of lemon or a big cinnamon stick into the pot.

NUTRITIONAL NOTE: Prunes are a good source of iron. Stewing them in an iron pot significantly increases the amount of iron they contain, and doesn't affect their flavor significantly.

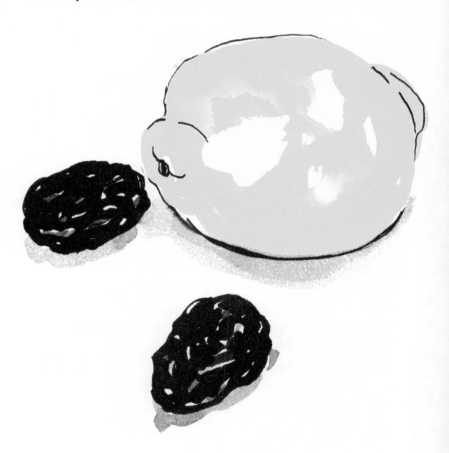

Best Bran Muffins

Need fiber? Try these *most* delicious muffins. Even the small size version boasts 2 tablespoons of bran each. Well worth eating even if you don't need extra fiber. In our community kitchen's copy of *The Laurel's Kitchen Bread Book,* the page with this recipe on it buckles, blotched with molasses stains. (Why just molasses? Some wag observed that *all* the ingredients you need for the recipe are right there on the page. Well, it saves on bookmarks.)

The recipe is sized to make 12 muffins in the pan with the smaller cup size, about ¼ cup each, 2¼″ across. If your pan has the larger, ½ cup size cups (2½″ across), double all the ingredients, and increase the cooking time by 5 minutes or so.

1 cup whole wheat flour
1 teaspoon baking soda
½ teaspoon salt
1½ cups wheat bran

3 tablespoons butter or oil
2 tablespoons brown sugar
2 tablespoons molasses
1 egg
1½ cups buttermilk

(½ cup raisins or currants)

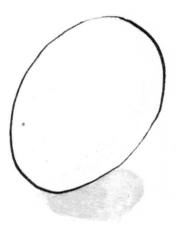

જે

Preheat oven to 375°F. Grease muffin pan.

Sift flour, soda, and salt together, and stir in the bran. Beat butter or oil and sugar and molasses together, and add the egg and buttermilk. Mix dry ingredients into liquids, adding raisins or currants if wanted. Place in the pan, filling the cups about ¾ full. Bake 15 to 20 minutes. Excellent.

You can bake these a few at a time. In flagrant violation of every rule about quick breads, the batter keeps fine for a week in the refrigerator and cooks up nicely.

An old trick to protect any muffin cups you don't have enough batter for, is to half fill them with hot water.

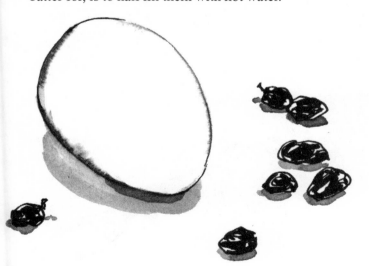

Good Noshes

Caregivers, how we wish there was always time for you to sit down and eat a leisurely meal in proper form! But sometimes it doesn't happen that way. Here are a few of our favorite pantry supplies for healthier snacking. Things will get better.

TOFU BARS

1 pound firm tofu
2 tablespoons soy sauce
2 tablespoons water

Good

Rinse tofu and slice crosswise into rectangular bars ¼″ to ½″ thick. Arrange slices in a greased 9″ x 13″ glass pan. Mix soy sauce and water, and pour over the tofu. Let stand an hour, if possible, shaking once or twice, or turning the tofu over at the halfway point.

Bake uncovered in a 325°F oven as long as an hour, until tofu is firm but not hard. It will become firmer as it cools. Store in the refrigerator and use to make sandwiches, or as a nibble.

You can add ginger, black pepper, curry powder, Mexican seasoning, or whatever you fancy, to the marinade.

There is much in the news these days about the benefits of eating soy. Anyway, sometimes a Tofu Bar works when you're looking for cheese, and that saves some calories and saturated fat. (Notice, though, the difference in calcium. Tofu varies in how much calcium it contains – check the label when you shop.)

3″ x 1¼″ x ¼″ piece	CALORIES	PROTEIN	TOTAL FAT	SAT.FAT	CALCIUM
Tofu Bar	54	6g	3.5g	0.5g	77mg
Jack cheese	106	7g	8.6g	5.4g	212mg

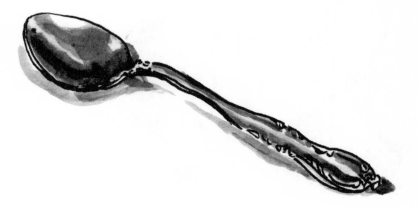

Cut vegetables of your choice into bite-size chunks and steam them just the way you like. Remove from pan and either dip in ice water, then drain well, or else spread them out in coldest place in your fridge. Salt and pepper, lemon juice or a little splash of good vinegar, if you like. Store covered in the refrigerator where you can reach them.

A surprisingly good variation on this theme: use zucchini, and toss while hot with a tiny bit of lemon and olive oil, then with salt, pepper, and grated Parmesan cheese to taste.

VEGETABLE BITES

*big head broccoli &
big head cauliflower*

*carrots, beets, asparagus,
green beans*

May sound weird, but awfully good nonetheless. When you bake yams for dinner, include a few extras, and keep them in the refrigerator. Good plain, eaten like fruit, or diced with celery, green peppers, lemon juice, and mayo for salad. Yams are high in complex carbohydrates, low in fat, and loaded with beneficial carotenes.

BAKED YAMS

Sometimes just keeping a bag of fresh mixed salad greens in the refrigerator is a very good ploy. The healthiest for sure, and among the tastiest of nibbles. Good rolled into a warm tortilla with a little salsa. Ai, arugula!

YUPPIE CHOW

Warm the small ones in the toaster, or directly over a gas burner, or on a griddle. Stuff them with combinations of cooked greens and salsa, with beans of course, with tofu or jack cheese and yuppie chow; with peanut butter and marmalade. In a pinch, one can even sprinkle a warm buttered tortilla with brown sugar and cinnamon. Tortillas keep for only about a week in the refrigerator, but they freeze well. Leave aside the white flour ones, most especially those made with lard. A normal corn tortilla has 67 calories, less than a gram of fat, and provides 52 mg of calcium.

TORTILLAS

Whole wheat bagels or pretzels; fruit of course, cherry tomatoes, popcorn, Smoothies, soup-in-a-cup (choose carefully), whole-grain low-fat crackers, brown rice crackers . . .

OTHER LOW-FAT SNACKS

Poppy Seed Noodles

¼ pound whole wheat ribbon noodles
¾ cups sour cream – regular, nonfat – or "Mock" (from any edition of Laurel's Kitchen)
1½ teaspoons poppy seeds
¼ teaspoon salt
(paprika)

A quick pasta dish to make while you steam the broccoli and cut up a big ripe tomato. Leftovers are good for lunch. Poppy Seed Noodles celebrate the warm flavor of whole wheat noodles; not so interesting when made with paler sorts.

If you have time to bake the casserole, preheat the oven to 350°F. Cook noodles in boiling, salted water until tender. Drain.

Combine all the ingredients; sprinkle with paprika and bake about 15 minutes in a greased 8″ square baking dish – or serve at once.

Makes 2 servings.

Instant Pizza

Toast one side of a slice of whole wheat bread, pocket bread, or an English muffin under the broiler. Turn over, and top with thick slices of red-ripe tomatoes or tomato sauce; sliced onion, peppers, steamed broccoli tops, mushrooms, etc., and top with any sort of grated cheese. Slide the pizza under the broiler until the cheese is melted. (Toaster ovens toast top and bottom at the same time.)

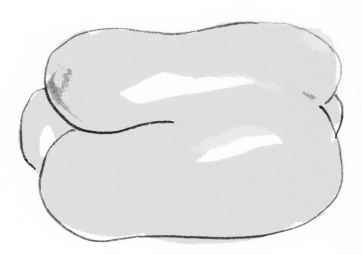

Baked Squash or Yams

These cook while you attend to other things. Their bright color tells you that they are packed with health-giving carotenes. Usually served with butter, but plenty good plain. (Honest! Just try them plain and see.)

Experiment with different varieties of yams. To tell the truth, what we call yams really are sweet potatoes, but whatever you call them, they elicit enthusiasm. We are partial to "Garnets," deep orange, extra sweet, and about right for one small serving. Regular potatoes can sit on the oven rack, but bake yams on a layer of kraft paper or chef's parchment set on a baking sheet, to protect your oven from the sugary drips. Garnets take about 45 minutes at 400°F; the big yams can take 2 hours. Done when soft.

Winter squash, all zillion kinds, are lower in calories than yams. Bake in serving-size chunks face down on a greased baking sheet, or in a glass baking pan with a half-inch of water in the bottom. A little brown sugar and cinnamon is fair, but more doesn't improve the flavor. Really, do try squash plain at least once, to taste the rich flavor!

Done when tender to your fork.

Bake extras, and use the rest to make Gingered Squash:

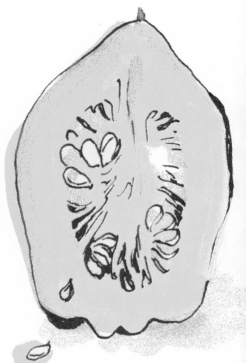

Gingered Squash

Our current top favorite way to serve squash. Digestible, fat-free, pretty. Leftovers excellent. (Butter is possible, but not necessary.)

&

Mix all ingredients, adjusting the amount of lemon and honey to balance the flavor – squashes vary a lot.

Makes about 1½ cups, 2 or 3 servings.

1½ cup hot, cooked winter
 squash, mashed
pinch salt
1 tablespoon minced or
 grated fresh gingerroot
juice of half a lemon
1 tablespoon honey
(1 tablespoon butter)

Creamy Green Soup

If you don't already know and love it, I guess it's possible that the idea might strike you as strange. Give it a try! Green soup appears frequently on our table in bowls or cups – it is one green dish that even green-allergic children truly welcome, in all its many versions.

Please note: You can use any leafy green vegetable to make green soup. But if you choose a member of the cole family (kale, collards, broccoli), keep the heat very gentle at all times.

৵০

PERFECTLY
HEAVENLY
3 cups milk
2 tablespoons butter
2 tablespoons flour (whole wheat pastry flour)
a very small onion
3 whole cloves
½ – ¾ teaspoon salt
dash nutmeg

1 bunch spinach (½ cup when cooked, drained, and chopped)

Warm milk in saucepan. In separate, heavy pan, melt butter and add flour; heat, stirring, a minute or so to cook the flour. Don't let it color. Add the milk and stir attentively while mixture comes to a boil and thickens.

Trim the onion. Remove and discard the heads of the cloves; stick the cloves into the onion and put it into the cream sauce. Add ½ teaspoon salt, and nutmeg. Set sauce over lowest possible heat, for half an hour if you have the time. Stir now and again to make sure it doesn't stick to the pan.

Wash spinach and cook lightly with just the water that clings to the leaves. Drain and chop.

Take the cloved onion out of the sauce and discard it. (Yep.) Blend spinach smooth with 1 cup of the sauce, then combine with the remaining sauce. Correct the seasonings – you may want more salt or nutmeg. Thin with more milk if a thinner soup is wanted. For best flavor serve warm, not piping hot. This lovely drink is soothing for anyone, sick or well, and good enough to serve on any occasion, even very fancy banquets.

৵০

CROCKPOT SOUP

Cook together: a quartered onion, 2 cloves garlic, a cup of well-rinsed green split peas, a big carrot, a giant handful of celery leaves, a bay leaf, a quartered potato, 1½ quarts of boiling water. When the peas and vegetables are all soft, remove the bay leaf and blend everything else. Add a scant teaspoon of salt, and pepper. Can add a spoonful of olive oil if you want to, also chopped parsley or basil. Check the salt. No need to blend if you chop the veggies, but this does make a delicious smooth blended soup.

Chop an onion and sauté in oil, adding a clove of garlic if you like. Add a couple of potatoes, cut into chunks, and water to cover. Cook until tender, then add a couple of quarts of washed, chopped spinach or chard. Simmer until greens are tender, then purée all of it. Add broth or milk to desired thick- or thinness, and salt and pepper to taste.

GREEN SOUP OF WINTER

As above, except only one potato, peeled please. Instead of the greens, add a pound and a half of cut-up asparagus and maybe half a dozen inner stalks of celery, including tender leaves, *finely chopped.*

SPRING GREEN SOUP

Chop and cook a couple of fresh, dark green zucchini with sautéed onion in enough broth or water to keep them from sticking. Blend smooth with the cooking liquid and a little butter; thin with milk, soymilk, buttermilk, or broth to drinking consistency. Our friend Francisco, who is five, helps prepare this recipe, and enjoys the soup, too. He likes to blend a spoon of cottage cheese into it.

SUMMER'S BOUNTY

Fresh zucchini straight from the garden, cooked and blended smooth with the cooking water. Serve in mugs with a dot of butter. Some like to stir in milk, soymilk, buttermilk.

SIMPLEST AND BEST

↤ *Good thinners:* Broth, milk, soymilk, buttermilk. Buttermilk is a wonderful flavor balancer and enhancer, but it has to be added at the end because when heated it tends to curdle. If that happens, return the soup to the blender. If a soup tastes "heavy" sometimes plain water is the gourmet addition.

MORE VARIABLES

↤ *Cut the fat:* Instead of sautéing the onion and garlic, boil them along with the other ingredients. The flavor is sweeter; some prefer it. Cook the onion thoroughly for best flavor.

↤ *Add* chopped basil or parsley, tiny green peas, corn off the cob. Serve with a dollop of salsa, yogurt, sour cream, hot herby croutons, or Parmesan or other grated cheese.

If you add cheese, grate it atop the individual servings. Should you put cheese in the pot with the soup it will coat the side of the pan in a way the dishwashing person will find hard to forgive.

TIP

Smoothies

The fastest meal. Blend sweet, soft fruit with equal amounts of buttermilk or yogurt, and milk. Additional sweetener is seldom necessary.

THE FRUITS

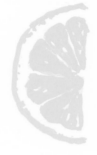

Banana, preferably perfectly ripe, stars in most smoothies because of its mellow sweetness and gift of thickening. In nonfat smoothies, the banana also counters chalkiness. Balance the flavor with something tart like buttermilk, yogurt, a slightly acidic fruit, a squeeze of lemon.

Strawberries make outstanding smoothies with peaches, bananas, with other kinds of berries, or solo.

Peaches and nectarines – terrific. Apricots too – though apricot smoothies need a banana, and even then you'll probably want to add some honey.

Blueberries, delicious, especially if you can appreciate attractive blue fleckiness.

ఎ

Bananas, because of their substantial peels, are generally free from pesticide residues. However, chemicals used on commercial plantations harm the workers, land, and water. Organic bananas taste much better.

The classic combination is a banana, a cut-up orange, plus a cup of yogurt or buttermilk, blended smooth.

Lemon can perk up a mixture that seems lackluster, but otherwise hold off using very acid fruits like plums or grapefruit unless you don't mind if the smoothie curdles.

Fruit juice (or concentrate) makes instant smoothies with yogurt or buttermilk, though you miss the freshness, and the valuable fiber. Apples don't work so well in smoothies, but apple juice plus buttermilk, with a dash of cinnamon, can be refreshing. A juice favorite is prune juice, a squeeze of lemon, and buttermilk: both tasty and therapeutic.

ఎ

If you get into smoothies, you will come up with endless combinations that please you as the seasons change. You can, of course, tailor your ingredients to address special needs. Smoothies are soothing for a patient who wants something cool, and they will please a child who otherwise would ask for ice cream. One mother we know freezes ripe bananas, peaches, or berries. With them she makes smoothies that satisfy her little boy's ice cream yearnings.

TAILORING

- ✧ *For more calories:* Blend in a tablespoon or two of almond or cashew butter – delicious additions – even peanut butter, for aficionados. Sometimes, use richer milk.
- ✧ *More calcium and protein:* A spoonful of skim milk powder increases calcium, protein, and other nutrients.
- ✧ *Minerals, B vitamins, protein:* A teaspoon nutritional yeast.
- ✧ *No dairy:* Use soymilk or fruit juice. Banana contributes texture and flavor to both of these.

VARIATIONS

You can freeze a smoothie and then give it a quick return trip to the blender or processor to make convincing frozen yogurt or *sorbet*. Commercial sorbets have superintense flavor; sorbet made from your average smoothie is more delicate. If you want intensity, make the smoothie with fruit juice concentrate straight from the can. Blend with banana, sweetener (if needed), and buttermilk or other "milk" to taste. Buttermilk blended with equal parts of lemon- or limeade concentrate is outrageously good. Horrific amounts of sugar, of course. Forget I mentioned it.

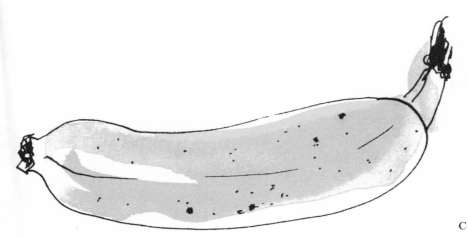

The Help You Need

I have been saving the best for last. Here is a caregiving tool effective in every situation; one you can start using right now. It can help you maintain élan under the most trying circumstances, including when you are just sitting there, waiting and watching.

This tool has many names because all great spiritual traditions have versions of it. From the earliest days, for example, Christians have called on the Name of Jesus, or repeated the Prayer of the Heart, "Lord Jesus Christ, have mercy on us." Muslims appeal to Allah in the tradition called *Al-Dhikr.* In Sanskrit, the term is *mantram* – "that which carries you across" – across the agitated mind, across the sea of life and death, across the next ten minutes. . . . Whatever you call them, this word or short phrase possesses tremendous power. Gandhi said, "The mantram becomes one's staff of life and carries one through every ordeal."

There are rules. You are supposed to choose one and stick to it, and repeat it in your mind as often as you can – really a lot. Like a journey of many similar steps, each repetition not only restores your focus and equilibrium, but brings you closer to your own best Self, the divine spark that glows in every heart.

Please choose one from your own religion, or else take Gandhi's mantram *Rama* (Raah-ma) – ancient, universal, one of the most beloved in the world. In times of stress, in times of despair, in times of soaring hopes, and when you are bored, repeat it in your mind. After a while, whenever things go badly, *Rama Rama* comes bubbling up to put them into perspective. When things go very well, *Rama Rama* reminds you not to let your mind fly out of control, heading for a crash. When you are angry, it cools you, and when you are fearful, it gently reassures. When you are lonely, it is a dear, fun, loyal friend that never leaves you. *Rama* makes waiting in line at the supermarket interesting, going to sleep sweeter than honey. Taking *Rama* for a walk is going hand in hand with joy. And, Dear Caregiver, when you sit quietly with your patient, holding *Rama* in your mind, it really will help both of you.

My heart goes out to every one of you. May your caregiving be a source of growth and joy for you, and solace for your patient.

Jesus, Jesus

Hail Mary

Allahu akbar

Barukh attah Adonai

Om mani padme hum

Rama

Om namah Shivaya

❧

In this space, I can only begin to tell you what the mantram can do. A lovely book about the Prayer of the Heart: The Way of a Pilgrim *written a century ago by a Russian peasant. For clear, detailed instructions, read* Meditation *(Nilgiri Press, 1993) or any other book by Eknath Easwaran.*

Index